The Penis Dialogues

Handle With Care

by

Gabriel Constans, Ph.D.

Aslan Publishing
Fairfield, CT

Aslan Publishing
2490 Black Rock Turnpike, #342
Fairfield, CT 06825
Please contact the publisher for a free catalog.
Phone: **203/372-0300**
Fax: **203/374-4766**
www.aslanpublishing.com

IMPORTANT NOTE TO READERS:

The information, examples annd suggestions in this book pertaining to physical and mental health, social relationships and sexual functioning are not meant to substitute for the advice of a licensed professional such as a medical doctor, psychiatrist or psychologist. The publishers and author expressly disclaim any liability for injuries resulting from use by readers of the ideas or methods contained herein.

Library of Congress Cataloging-in-Publication Data

Constans, Gabriel.
The penis dialogues : handle with care / by Gabriel Constans.
p. cm.
Includes bibliographical references.
ISBN 0-944031-94-3
1. Penis. 2. Masculinity, 3. Men--Sexual behavior. 4. Penis--Social aspects. 5. Penis--Physiology. I. Title

GT498.P45C66 2003
3-5.31--dc22

2003058257

Editing and book design by Dianne Schilling
Cover design by Miggs Burroughs
Author photo by Shona Constans Blumeneau
Printing by Baker Johnson, Inc.
Printed in the USA

"*The Penis Dialogues: Handle with Care* is a pioneering work. Men's feelings and attitudes about their sexuality, gender and experiences of being male have seldom been spoken of with such honesty and insight. Read this book!"

Bob Stahl, Ph.D.
Director of Stress Reduction Program

"Gabriel Constans has created a heads up, hands-on exploration of the male member. It is both amusing and informative."

James McElheron
Building Consultant and Supervisor

"This book has started a dialogue that we will continue with the men and women in our lives. I predict that you, too, will start asking others some of the questions the author has posed. I hope the penis dialogues have only just begun."

Elizabeth Sparks
Videographer and Historian

"Rarely have men's relationships to their bodies and sexuality been so enlightening and entertaining. It's not often that a book arrives on the scene that comes in so handy."

Bruce Hobson, Health Educator

"*The Penis Dialogues: Handle with Care* gives voice, with vulnerable honesty, to the experience of male sensuality and sexuality. Read it with care. The opportunity for deeper understanding and healing for both men and women alike is woven throughout this book."

Jan Landry, Chaplain

"I was struck by this book's humor, probing curiosity and genuine compassion."

Eve Ensler, Playwright
Author of *The Vagina Monologues*

Dedication

To all the men of the world who are rediscovering their bodies and desires with conscious concern, caring and commitment—journeying beyond media labels, cultural conditioning and social expectations. May we continue to embrace our sexuality in all its magnificent manifestations, and love our partners and ourselves with passion, creativity and tenderness.

Acknowledgements

It is with deep appreciation and gratitude that I thank Eve Ensler for listening to women's stories and experiences and having the courage and tenacity to create, perform and write *The Vagina Monologues*. We are all, male and female, indebted to her insightful observations and willingness to present the joyful, humorous, degrading and painful realities women around the world live with every day.

Ms. Ensler has brought the human condition to light, in both its glory and suffering and helped women discover and re-claim their sexuality, wisdom, individuality, strength and creative spirit.

I hope *The Penis Dialogues: Handle With Care* will impact men's lives in the same way.

The women's movement, both past and present, has provided the people of this world the opportunity to move beyond stereotypes, constraints and limitations. Women have been our explorers and have taught men how to be free human beings. Blessings to you all.

Without the loving guidance and support of the folks at Aslan Publishing this book would not be in its present form. Another publisher might have squeezed it into a cliché and marketed it as a sex or humor book. Barbara Hoberman Levine immediately understood my intentions and helped guide these stories, facts and insights about men to fruition. I could feel receptivity, encouragement and excitement flow from her home on the East Coast to mine on the West. Many thanks to other members of the Aslan team: Dianne Schilling for her skillful editing, and Miggs Burroughs for his creative cover design.

To all the men who took the risk and the time to speak with me about their bodies, thoughts, feelings and experiences, thank you. Your generosity, integrity and clarity were unexpected, overwhelming and enlightening. You have my respect and admiration for walking this journey and being "man enough" to honestly acknowledge your pain, fears, regrets, joys, pleasures, frustrations, hopes and dreams.

Contents

Interview Questions

Introduction

I talked with hundreds of men. Young and old men; brothers, fathers, sons, grandfathers and uncles; heterosexual, homosexual and bisexual men; black, brown and white men; rich and poor men; short, tall, round and thin men; doctors, farm-workers, teachers, roofers, executives, counselors, tile-layers, college students, carpenters, stay-at-home dads and men who are unemployed.

We met at men's groups, in sports bars, on the bus, at conferences, in private homes, at baseball games, parties, concerts and bowling leagues. We talked alone or in small groups. Our contacts were in person, through the Internet or by phone.

We talked about the penis in ways men seldom, if ever, have before. We explored its effects upon our lives and how being male is experienced and perceived. We spoke beyond the clichés, the jokes and comparisons of male virility and power. We spoke from our hearts with honesty, curiosity, shock, bemusement and surprise.

The Penis Dialogues is not about judging, manipulating or reinforcing inequality and power in our relationships; it is not about being "better" or "worse" than another. You won't find tales of sexual exploits presented to titillate, or to boast about being macho, though sexual experiences are openly discussed.

The purpose of this book is to assist men to find common ground and to celebrate their differences and similarities. It is about identifying and choosing to break free of thousands of years of cultural conditioning and stereotyping that keeps men separated from one another and from the opposite sex. It investigates and lays bare the facts, myths, experiences, misperceptions and stories of that member of the male body that is held so dear and by which men so often are defined.

Whether you read *The Penis Dialogues* for entertainment, pleasure, education, enlightenment or simple curiosity, please—handle with care.

If Your Penis Could Talk

The Agony and the Ecstasy

I was told that my life started out with a close call. Not long after coming into this world they pulled back my skin and cut off the protective lining that covered my head just a few millimeters from the end of my urethra. Can you imagine?! They didn't ask me what I thought about it, just stretched it out and whack! Thank God I was just a little tyke then and don't remember the trauma. I was informed that it was a bloody mess and took a week to heal.

The next thing I recall was sitting in the warm bathtub, with the six-year-old boy to whom I am intimately attached. He and his younger sister would pull my foreskin up over my head and push me as deep inside of him as I would go. He would carefully hold me back as they both counted. "Ten, nine, eight, seven, six, five, four, three, two, one, zero, blast off!" At zero he would let go. They both laughed and giggled hysterically as I shyly emerged and floated to the surface.

It wasn't long afterwards that I occasionally felt my skin being touched in a most pleasurable way. On those occasions, my pores became engorged and I filled up with blood. Then something rumbled deep inside me and a flood of liquid erupted through my opening. The body I was attached to had grown into a young man and he'd discovered that I was useful for something besides going pee.

I recall a most embarrassing time when he and a young woman, both fully clothed, where in a dark room kissing and touching. I guess he had never felt a girl so closely and was so excited that he couldn't stop the flood that wet his pants. Somehow he hid the spot until we got home and changed. He'd have been mortified if anyone noticed.

The next memory I have is a painful incident involving a horse. My young man and I were out in a field innocently standing in front of his horse Stanley. He was petting the horse's nose, when another big horse approached. Without any warning Stanley reared up and kicked with its front hooves towards the stallion standing behind us. Needless to say, we were caught right in between.

A searing pain shot through me and my boy's contracted testicles—my closest relatives. We reacted with such ferocity that we thought we had retreated into his stomach cavity. He fell to the ground, curled up in agony, unable to speak or move.

The horses didn't step on us and someone who had seen what happened came running to help. They carried us inside, where we lay with ice bags for two to three days until the swelling, discoloration and extreme agony subsided. Luckily, there was no permanent damage, other than a life-long fear of horses.

Not long after that calamity came a bout of extended ecstasy when we had our first love affair and sexual encounter with another human being.

After much apprehension, preparation and excitement, I found myself inside the warm, wet walls of his girlfriend. We were sixteen years old at the time. Thank goodness she knew what she was doing, because he didn't have a clue. The minute he entered that soft, hot, enfolding cave of pleasure, his juices burst through me like a flood. There was no way he could hold back. I heard her say, "That's OK, just wait a few minutes and we'll do it again."

Damn, if she wasn't right. It only seemed like seconds and I was as hard as a fat carrot being thrust in and out of her vagina with increasing speed, force and passion. When he came a second time, so did she. The mixture of her waters and undulating muscles and his river of fluids was the closest thing to heaven that we'd ever known.

A few years have passed since those highs and lows. We're in our mid-forties now. He's had a few love affairs here and there, a painful operation or two, and helped to create a number of children. I continue to be used for basic necessities and for pleasure, both alone and with his wonderful partner, whom he calls his best friend and wife. In spite of all the ups and downs and ins and outs, I wouldn't have wanted to be attached to any other guy.

PENIS FACTS

The Male of the Chicken

In Latin *penis* (pes) means tail. The dictionary defines it as, "The male organ of sexual intercourse: in mammals it is also the organ through which urine is ejected."

The dictionary describes the word *cock* as:

- the male of the chicken
- the male of other birds
- the crowing of a rooster
- a weather vane in the shape of a rooster
- a leader or chief, especially one with some boldness or arrogance
- a faucet or valve for regulating the flow of a liquid or gas
- a tilting or turning upward
- a jaunty, erect position
- to set; to be ready for release
- a small, cone-shaped pile.

I don't believe I've ever thought of my cock as a "cone-shaped pile" or an "arrogant leader or chief." Nor have I thought of an erection as "jaunty," but I guess I'll have to reconsider. After all, these facts are in the dictionary as plain as day and who am I to question Webster's?

1

What's in a Name?

What labels, terms of endearment, derogatory slang or pet names have you or someone else given your penis?

Prick
Dick
Pecker
Rod
Staff
Cock
Willie
Schlong
Dong
Mr. Happy
Peacemaker
Joy Stick
Mr. Flipper

The Unit
Anteater
Thing
Dillie-What
Houdini
Hard Candy
Vegra
Traveler
Pet
Precious
Hard Drive
My Business
Mack
My Munchie
Carrot
Dog
Hotdog
Salami
Pack
Bean Shooter
Baby Maker
Seed Planter
Percy
Henry
Dink
Big Will
Big Guy
Woody
Weenie
Weiner
Na-na
Manhood
Middle Leg
Shaft

Chicken
Bald-headed Monkey
Pito
Leno
Firewood
The Quarterback
Big Foot
The Pussy Duster
Frankie
Come Doctor
Swelled Head
Member
Jones
My Microphone
Mambo
Prowler
Diver Swimmer
Love Machine
The Incredible Heat- Seeking Moisture Missile
Lilly
Wedding Tackle
Todger
Dober
Prowler
Wally
Johnson
Lizard
Pouch
Basket
Family Jewels
Meat and Potatoes
Hap-penis
Wang
Wanger

Wacker
One-Eyed Ring-Neck Trouser Snake
Porpoise
The Big Stick
Bird
Bottom Rocker
Bulldog
Chub
Gila Monster
Love Pump
Peni
Phallus
Porky
Pride and Joy
Privates
Throber
Magic Wand

If Your Penis Could Talk

Don't Look a Gift Horse in the Mouth

My man and I had just turned eighteen. All we'd been thinking about for years was sex, sex, sex and more sex. I was hard so often it's a wonder I didn't burst. I don't know how he walked around half the time without me bumping into something and hurting us.

It seemed like everyone else we knew had gotten laid, had sex, screwed, whatever you want to call it, except us. Then we hit pay dirt.

About a month ago we were at an all-night Keg with some friends. My guy was drinking beer, listening to music and just kicking back. He and his buddies had graduated from high school a few weeks earlier and some of them were going off to college in the city.

My man and I were staying home on the ranch and figured we wouldn't see any women or get a piece of ass until we got married or something. There weren't many women around these parts and the ones we knew were all taken or gone.

Well, he was just sitting there, me dangling between his bony old knees, when his friend Samuel arrived in his truck and walked in with these two hot looking chicks.

"Where the hell did he find them?" My guy wondered.

Samuel said, "I brought you guys a present. It's all on me. This here is Julia." He squeezed the brunette around the shoulders. "And this fine lady is Bunny." He gave her a wink.

They were old, about mid-thirties, but they looked real good.

At first we didn't realize what he was saying, then it slowly dawned on my guy. There are four of us, counting Samuel, and now these two women. We didn't realize they were hookers until Conrad tried to hand Samuel some money and Sam shook his head no and said, "I told you it's on me."

Well, it seemed like we'd been waiting for this all our lives and now that it was about to happen we were as nervous as a spooked steer.

Samuel asked the fellas who'd like to go first and which girl they wanted. Conrad jumped right up and went to Bunny. She put her arms around him and they started going at it.

Samuel said, "I'll hang with Julia. Why don't you guys wait outside? He nodded at Jim and us.

We acted real cool, like we'd done this a thousand times and went outside. We started pacing back and forth, trying not to listen, but it was impossible to block out their moaning. I start getting a real hard-on. My guy and Jim didn't look at each other, but it seemed like Jim and his cock were just as nervous.

When Samuel opened the door and waved us in, he and Conrad had big stupid grins on their faces and the girls were buck-naked.

As soon as Conrad and Samuel left, Julia started unbuttoning my man's pants and Bunny took off Jim's. Before I knew what was happening I was experiencing the sweetest sensations I'd ever known. Julia was gently sucking me and my guy was closing his eyes and loving it.

It was only a minute or two before I felt like I was going to cream. I heard her say, "Slow down boy. Take your time." That stopped us for a minute or two, but that was about all. The pleasure was just too awesome and we came all over the place.

My guy glanced over at Jim and Bunny and saw that they were still going at it strong. Jim was screwing her from behind and she was yelling like she loved it. He looked over at us and saw my man pulling up his pants and tucking me inside.

Suddenly, my guy seemed to be embarrassed or something and wanted to run away. He looked at Julia and said, "Sorry," then high-stepped it out of the cabin all the way to the county road.

Sam picked us up later, with Jim, Conrad and the girls in the back of the truck and asked my guy, "What gives?"

He just said, "Nothing." I figure he felt that no matter how good it was, the real thing didn't measure up to the anticipation. I think he also felt a little bad about paying somebody for something that he thought should come naturally with someone he had feelings for, but he didn't want to wimp out with his friends and act like a pussy.

PENIS FACTS

Egyptian King's Divine Erection

Images of Min (also known as Menu, Khem and Amsu) have been found in Egyptian artifacts dating back to 3,000 B.C. He was usually portrayed with a large erect penis and worshiped as a god of virility, sexual prowess and fertility.

His image and cultural influence penetrated much of the known world of the time and spawned the creation of Cupid, Dionysius, Bacchus and Pan in Asia-Minor and Europe. But of all the male gods of love that followed, none was as forthright or unambiguous about his sexuality as Min.

During the days of Min it was believed that one's sexual life was holy. The Egyptians and surrounding peoples viewed sex as a personal and social human connection to the divine.

Min was more than a myth. He was a real man known as King Menes or The Scorpion King and was the first known Pharaoh of Egypt. He united both the lower and upper regions of the country and was known for his sexual stamina and exploits as the "eternally firm" king.

Min brought his Sumerian language with him when he arrived in Egypt from Sumer. Egyptian hieroglyphics were derived from the Sumerian dialect. He greatly valued artistic creation and expression and was the first to construct public buildings and temples for all the people of the area.

If Your Penis Could Talk

World Cup Climaxes with Family Jewels

I've been around the world a time or two and had a splendid time of it. I was stuck in the pants of a military uniform for over twenty years and traveled to every continent. I've been on boats, planes, motorcycles, cars, helicopters, tanks and trains.

In every country we visited I was let out to play. From my perspective sex seemed the same in any language.

Though the women I entered spoke different languages, their pussies were warmly familiar, yet unique. Some were wide and welcoming and some were tight and narrow. Others were dripping wet and some barely moist. They all felt wonderful to me. The excitement, anticipation and release were top rate. I have no complaints, regrets or guilt.

After years of living around the globe, my man and I settled down, got married and helped produce two children. It was quite a contrast to the life we had lived, but his wife said she loved him and, though it became monotonous after a while, we had sex frequently enough to keep him domesticated and at home. He even got a job in the private sector and liked it.

About five years after the second child was born, his wife got fed up with the various birth control methods and insisted that he get a vasectomy. I had no idea what that was, but soon found out.

One afternoon, after the tubes in his testicles were severed, we were lying on the cot packed in ice (so we wouldn't swell). He had his coffee, TV controller, paper—everything he needed on the bedside table.

We were just settling down when his kids got home from school and came running into the room yelling, "Daddy Daddy!" They jumped directly onto the bed.

We hit the ceiling! It hurt like, well . . . like my man's testicles had been stabbed with a knife.

It's not a pleasant memory and we've taken great pains to forget it.

PENIS FACTS

What Did You Say?

In German cock is *hahn*. In French it is *coq*. In Spanish it is *grifo*. And in Chinese cock is *xiong ji*.

To call a penis a cock or prick was common in the 17th century. Jock and Jack have also meant the penis since the 16th century, both coming from the familiar names for John. Dick became a common name for the penis around the time of the American Civil War.

If Jock and Jack originated from John, and mean the same thing as Dick, why don't we call people a penis, a john or a jack when we refer to someone we don't like or are angry at? I guess it doesn't have quite the same ring to say, "You john" or "Quit being such a penis."

When did calling someone the male organ become derogatory? Such a functional and pleasurable part of the anatomy doesn't seem to satisfy the desire to put someone down. Calling someone a dick or a pussy seems like it should be a compliment instead of slander. And saying someone or something "sucks" to mean it's bad doesn't make sense either. Sucking or being sucked feels great. How did it come to mean the opposite?

2

Dancing in the Spotlight

What does your penis look like or remind you of?

Author's note: *This was one of the few questions that men seemed reluctant to answer, yet it received some of the biggest laughs when they finally did. A man's age didn't seem to have any bearing on his apprehension. The anxiety surrounding the question may have signaled fear. Fear of what others would think, fear of judgment, or comparisons, or of not appearing "normal."*

Though an abundance of romantic and eroticised images of the male organ appear in art, religion and various cultural traditions throughout the ages, it seems that present day man has little regard for the penis as an object to be admired or as a symbol of creation. Men tend to refer to the penis as a simple tool, or thing, and compare it to animals or food. Here are a few of their more revealing replies.

It reminds me of Winston Churchill with a cigar.

This reminds me of a Cheech and Chong joke. "I'm circumcised, but I'm also circumscribed." But . . . if you really want to know . . . the glandular part of my head is impressive. I'm of average length when I'm erect and thick. My penis is darker than the rest of my body and looks like it has a suntan. It reminds me of Moses' staff. Moses had a big stick that did tricks. It's a dumb fellow, this stick. It needs another member to talk for it.

When it's soft it reminds me of a mole.

When it's hanging it reminds me of a cross between a guinea pig and Humpty Dumpty. If it's erect it's like a silver baton.

Most of the time I'm just grateful to have something to hang onto. When you're in your later fifties, you pee a lot more than you have sex. It's like my thumb, my elbow and my left ear; it's just another strange part of my body.

It reminds me of a cobra that's been aroused and is waiting to strike. It rises, flares up and sways back and forth.

It looks ugly. I think it's smaller than average, but most guys think theirs is bigger or smaller than everyone else's anyway. When it's drooping, it reminds me of a slug.

It depends what day it is. Sometimes it reminds me of a partly filled sausage container. It's like the trunk of a tree. It moves, changes or adapts its personality to the environment. It's malleable.

An extra thumb.

Answering this question makes me realize it's not just a utilitarian device. It is more like an expression of self, more than a thing or object that has a fixed imprint of its own. It's directly reflective of how I partly see myself, whereas my nostrils or earlobes aren't.

My penis looks like a small, friendly version of a sea cucumber. The sea cucumber looks like the penis of the sea. And then again, sometimes it looks like a bird without feathers.

It sort of looks like a shriveled up finger. There are many things that remind me of the penis, especially male and female plugs in plumbing, and nuts and screws.

When asked by a colleague, "Do you think a person's self-image is dependent on the size of his penis?" Sigmund Freud answered, "It is quite the opposite. The size of his penis depends on his self-image."

It looks like a piece of meat. Symbolically it has a lot of history; it's like my historical root. It has been so much a part of the human condition and is represented in many cultures and rituals.

It reminds me of a well-shaped zucchini when it's erect.

It looks like a little fireman. It's got a round hat with a rim around the top. When it's erect it's all smooth, shiny and pulsating and when it's not it's like a little shriveled worm with wrinkled skin. Sometimes it seems like a miracle when it gets hard and quadruples in size.

3

A Woman's Eyeview

What does a penis look like to you?

Author's note: *Women don't seem to see the penis much differently than men—most of the time. Their images and descriptions are quite similar, though a few comments caught me with my pants down.*

It looks like an elephant seal. I wouldn't want one. I think women are prettier.

Flaccid, it looks like a sleeping worm. Erect it looks silly.

Like a rocket or missile.

A dildo or a tree on a deserted island.

It reminds me of a cactus, a flesh-colored flower or an umbrella.

It must be difficult to walk around with one when its erect.

When it's soft it looks like a package, combined with testicles.

It's like a magic wand, a hairless wonder or a Sergeant Major.

They're pretty, soft, hard, shriveled and attached.

The Seattle space needle.

Like a windsock at the airport without any air in it and when it's erect it looks like a pole.

Erect, it looks like a tall candle that's melted in the sun and bends slightly. It also reminds me of the Empire State Building.

Flaccid, it looks like a little Gherkin pickle.

A fire hydrant.

A dangly thing, like a dangling participle.

There's nothing else that looks like it.

They look shiny.

It's pink and hard.

It's just a sticky-outy thing.

A penis is a one-eyed snake.

When it's down it looks like a willow tree.

It looks sort of funny and makes me wonder what it's

like to have one. It's just a fleshy thing that hangs there. It doesn't make much of an impression on me.

Like a mushroom.

Have you ever seen a banana? Well . . .

It looks like a balloon with a lot of hot air in it.

If it's soft it looks like a turnip. If it's hard it looks like a zucchini.

It's similar to a pointed pencil or ruler that the teacher is always pointing at you, telling you to do this or that.

It reminds me of a beautiful cactus, without thorns, that holds life-quenching water in its roots.

It always reminds me of water fountains and those statues in Europe with little boys peeing into the pond.

They're like a small, firm hand-warmer when they're erect and snuggled up against your back

If Your Penis Could Talk

Blowing His Top

The first several times Jerry and I had sex with his new girlfriend he would always make me pull out at the last minute and take random shots at the headboard, her armpit or whatever was close by. They both wanted to make sure none of those little sperm that flew through my subway met up with any ripe old eggs at the end of the tunnel. It was very frustrating for Jerry, let alone me. Staying inside for those last couple of squeezes always feels so wonderful.

One night, when they were going real hot and heavy they decided to use a condom so Jerry wouldn't have to pull out, and covered me up with this rubbery thing. Well, wouldn't you know it, the first time they dressed me up the top of the condom tore off. I swear I had nothing to do with it. I was just doing my thing.

When I finally pulled out Jerry said, "Oh my God, you won't believe what happened." They both looked down. The top of the condom was nowhere in sight. I had a great time breaking free, but they had to deal with the possible consequences.

PENIS FACTS

Lost in Space

After reaching puberty the testicles continuously produce about 200 million sperm a day. Most men ejaculate about 5000 times during their adult lives, which equals approximately 1 trillion sperm produced and discharged in a man's lifetime.

Is it any wonder that we are so exhausted, or fall asleep after orgasm, or die on average years before women? We're used up, wrung out and sucked dry. Is it worth it? Definitely. But wouldn't it have been easier to have us produce just one or two super strong, healthy sperm at a time instead of wasting so much energy on millions of duds that perish in route or end up in the wrong space?

If Your Penis Could Talk

Running for My Life

The guy I'm attached to is named Ricky. Five days a week during his freshman days at college, he'd stuff me inside this thing called a jockstrap and put a hard plastic thing, called a cup, over me. Then he'd slip into these tight-ass pants and put on shoulder pads, a helmet and other kinds of protective devices.

Then he'd run out of the locker room with a bunch of other guys, yelling and screaming, with all their cocks crammed into these cups. I couldn't see where we were going or what was going on, but I could hear a lot of hollering, grunting and swearing.

He told me they were practicing something called football and all the stuff around me was for my own good. Maybe so, but I missed my free-swinging freedom for the rest of the day and night and resented being cooped up like a jack-in-the-box.

Once a week, when they played against another team, Ricky and these guys would play extra hard. It was usually Saturday night, one of my favorite times to be out looking around, but I sure as hell wasn't about to come out at a time like this.

Ricky was moving forward, backwards and sideways. I was trying to keep up and readjust myself to the lay of the land, so to speak, when somebody yells at him, "Run Ricky. Run like hell."

Ricky had something in his hands and was running so fast, I thought I'd be bounced to death. Then, out of nowhere, we got hit head on. And I mean head on. Some guy from the opposite team must have lowered his head and hit Ricky in the groin with his helmet, because the next thing I knew I was trying to climb up his gut, along with his balls, and we were lying on the ground in agony.

"Hey!" I screamed. "I thought all this stuff around me was supposed to make this safe! I thought we were protected! What's going on?!"

Ricky must have thought the same thing. He seemed just as surprised as I was. I don't think he held on to the football—they called it a fumble—and at that point he didn't care what else was going on.

He just wanted the shooting pains to stop and to have me back where I belonged with my testicle friends.

The coaches took us to the sideline, surrounded us with players so the people in the stands couldn't see, and started massaging Ricky's lower stomach until we came back down. Then they put some ice between his legs, which was another shock, but it helped prevent me from swelling.

After the first half was over and we reconnoitered in the locker room, he stuffed me back in the so-called protective cup and like an idiot went running out screaming again. I was just hanging in their wondering, "Is this guy crazy?"

4

It Feels So Good

When did you first discover that touching your penis felt good, and what were you told about masturbation?

Author's note: *Since our society is becoming increasingly sexually liberated, I expected a significant portion of the men I interviewed to have been told about masturbation by their parents. But regardless of age or generation, the majority had been told zilch about the pleasures and benefits of self-gratification. It seems that the fathers and mothers of these men were just as squeamish, embarrassed or ill-prepared to talk about masturbation as were their parents and grandparents. This reality led most of the men to discover the fine art of self-gratification by word-of-mouth or solo experimentation.*

I remember pulling myself along in a crib and feeling this wonderful rubbing sensation underneath. I must have been pre-verbal, but the memory stayed with me.

The first time I can recall noticing that touching myself felt good was in a preschool. It was a Sunday-school nursery and my parents were in church. I was rocking in a three-dimensional swan and it was really, really good. It was just the best swan. I think it gave me an orgasm, though I couldn't ejaculate that young.

It was a lot later for me than most guys. I think I was around nine or ten. I was lying on my stomach in bed and for some reason I suddenly become aware of my penis pressed between the mattress and my stomach. It was sensitive and pleasurable. I soon started touching myself all the time and remember feeling sore after a week or two from doing it so much. My Dad once said, somewhat awkwardly, "The things you hear about masturbation aren't true. You won't go blind."

I must have been about two or three years old. I watched my own two sons start to become aware that touching themselves felt good right around the same age. Obviously nobody told them what to do, they just discovered it on their own. It seemed instinctual. When I was young my brothers and I would play Aztec sacrifice. It was a game where we would touch each other's penis and say, "Rise."

I joined the Mormon Church when I was sixteen, so enjoying myself through masturbation was put on hold for a long time. I joined at the time because my father was a violent alcoholic and I wanted to be with men who claimed to have it together and didn't act like he did.The fallout was that I received a set of doctrinal pamphlets on how I should conduct my sexuality, which was essentially based on shame. When I realized that such an extreme view of guilt was totally out of whack, I began to fully enjoy the art of self-pleasuring. I believe now that if I had not gone through the Mormon indoctrination, and waited so long, I might not have enjoyed masturbation and sex as much as I did later in life. The long abstinence made it sweeter. I owe it to Mr. Mambo (my cock) for making me an "evil person."

When I was about fourteen I discovered a book in my parents bedside table that had photographs of different sexual positions. I snuck into the bathroom, looked at the pictures and felt myself get hard. I kept looking at the pictures and stroking and rubbing myself. Eventually there was a slow leakage, but no ejaculation. It was my first sense of my penis being an instrument I could play. My whole world opened up and I discovered that my penis was good for something besides peeing. After that I began to do it frequently and was very keen to try it with women.

The first time I had an orgasm I woke up and realized I'd been stroking myself against the pillow and had made a mess in my sleeping bag. I thought this was really weird, but I liked it. I wondered if what had happened was OK and if the nuns or priests had somehow seen me. Even as an adult I feel like someone's looking over my shoulder.

When I was seven I felt a strong sexual feeling that went from my thighs all the way up to my head. I was in the backyard. My grandfather, an inventor, had made a telescope for our family. It was a pale green, four-foot long cylinder aimed towards the sky. I climbed up on top of it, slid down and felt something happen. I did it again and the same thing happened. I went into the house and told my mother, "I slid down the telescope and it made me feel dizzy, funny and good." She said, "Well, be careful you don't fall." When I got older I read every sex book I could get my hands on, away from home, and became a fountain of information for my group of friends.

My brother and I had bunk beds. He had the top and I was below. One night, when the two of us were about six, we started playing with each other's penis like they were toys. Just as I told him, "Faster, faster." my father walked in and said, "OK, cut it out. It's time to go to sleep."

A friend and I went up into our tree house. He was jacking off and I said, "What are you doing?" He told me and

I said, "I've never done that before." He said, "Do you want to do that with me?" I did it to him, then tried it with myself. When I came, it was a complete surprise. I had no idea such an incredible thing could happen. It was like having a new friend, going to a new place or being told an incredible secret. I just thought it was a normal thing for people to do. There was some negative morality around it growing up. Most of it came from religious and cultural biases, both Catholic and Jewish.

My Mom took me to a pediatrician and, without telling me why, left me alone in the room with him. He took out a chart of the body and said if I was in a dark alley with a woman to keep my pants zipped. That was the only sex education I received.

When I was about four years old another boy showed me how to play "nasty." It was the first time I knew what an erection was—such as it was at four. Then, when I was ten years old, another boy showed me how to masturbate and told me to keep doing it until it felt good. It took a long time, but it worked. I remember a big guy at camp inspecting our penises when we went to the lake. He asked me once if I was playing with it. I said, "No." He said, "Good. Don't start."

I was in junior high school when a kid in the men's locker room told me that if you rubbed your penis it would feel good. Later that week, at home, I tried it out and had my first orgasm. I was familiar with erections, as I had them a lot, but I didn't really understand them. I had never known the part about rubbing it when it was hard. When I did, it was a wonderful surprise to have an orgasm. It was strange and a bit scary, but it felt so good. The end of my penis would vibrate and all this liquid came out. I didn't know what to do with it. It was like I was making a breakthrough in science, a new discovery. At the time, I thought I should hide my discovery. It felt shameful, but oh so good.

When I reached high school my dad told me about

babies in a unique sort of way. He took me to the Safeway parking lot in his Chevy, scrunched over the steering wheel and mumbled a bunch of stuff I could hardly hear. What I did hear was very clinical. He was very uncomfortable and looked like he just wanted to get it all over with. He must have mumbled at that dashboard for at least two minutes, then we left.

I roughly recall that early in my life it felt good to scratch and rub down there. It gave me a sense of connection and wholeness that swiping at a baseball and missing just didn't produce. The scratching and rubbing felt like self-cultivation, like I was raking my private garden and making things grow. My parents said nothing. I read a Boy Scout manual once that had several paragraphs about wet dreams.

My mother was a super Catholic and I went to Catholic schools most of my life, so there was a lot of taboo about sex. I started masturbating at about fifteen. Masturbating felt like intense anticipation and wanting to stick this thing somewhere and come—like something better is on the horizon. It was psychological as well as physical. My early erections were usually accompanied by embarrassment because they occurred at times when I was around a lot of other kids and I was afraid someone would look at my pants and make fun of me. I also had an irrational and exaggerated fear about nudity. The first erection I had was accompanied by the fear that my pants would fall off or someone would disrobe me and make me naked. All of my experience as a young man was influenced by my mother, whose mother never told her anything about sex and wouldn't even utter the word "pregnant" in front of her children, even though she had six.

I was never told anything by my parents. Everything around sex was considered dirty. Now I think masturbation is great and healthy. I was finally able to come to terms with the guilt instilled in me as a young man and let it go.

I was about ten when I discovered that it felt good to

touch myself. It happened during the usual games with the neighborhood kids. Kids saying, "Can I see yours?" and "I'll show you mine." My father explicitly told me that masturbation was not a bad thing.

In *my* days—I'm seventy now—the most common thing told us about masturbation was that if you did it you would get "blue balls." That meant your testicles would swell up, you couldn't walk and you would have to go see a doctor. It was also common knowledge, at the time, that masturbation could make you grow crazy.

When I was about twelve my Mom ripped off the covers of my bed and saw that I had a hard-on. She noticed right away and said something about it being a sin. When I was twenty my Dad said, "Make sure to use condoms." That was all they ever said about it.

I was at my neighbor's house. He was two years older than I was. I remember it clearly. He had a magazine with pictures. If I close my eyes I can still see those pictures. He was telling me about jacking-off and started doing it. I started touching myself and thinking, "Wow, does this feel good!" It was all so new. When I had an orgasm I looked down and wondered, "What's all this white stuff?" My parents didn't tell me anything about it and sex education at school never talked about masturbation.

My parents were heavy-duty Protestants. They didn't even talk about toilet paper. When I was fourteen we went to Europe where there were a number of nude statues. My Dad took me around and showed me the young people, then showed me the older men in the statues and quickly turned away.

Nobody said anything about masturbation or the birds and bees when I was young. My Dad gave me a lecture and all he said was, "Keep your wiener in your pants." That was it. He was so embarrassed.

If Your Penis Could Talk

Free Willy!

No more interference from that big head on top of those shoulders. Now I'm in charge and we're going for the whole enchilada. No more confinement inside those sweaty, tight pants. I want to feel a warm breeze moving across my head and rustling the hair on my balls. Freedom—that's where real living awaits. Peeing where and when I want without feeling restricted or confined. Not caring whether I drip or dribble, I'm in charge now. I AM PENIS, HEAR ME ROAR!

Phew...having said that, I feel much better. Actually I don't really like being outside very much, shrinkage and all, except when there is a fire that needs putting out. Then I'm Johnny Johnson the Fireman, on the spot, ready and willing to lend a helping hand. Since the helping hand is one of my best friends, I'm always ready to assist whenever needed. Unfortunately, this is where I usually have problems with the big guy upstairs. He's got all kinds of issues that really screw me up causing me to perk up when there is absolutely no chance of action, and then go limp when the promised land is in sight! Whoa, how confusing is that. If his head were as focused as mine, then life would be great.

It's not easy being a penis these days, especially if you're just a regular guy. The pressures for conformity are getting worse, too. Between all the new diseases, the man-eating women, and the men who somehow think men are women, it's confusing to say the least. Things are getting better though. There's talk of marriage between the big guy and a very cute woman. Actually, this means nothing to me except the distinct possibility of regular action. Yea baby, the drought is over and I do believe the best is yet to cum.

PENIS FACTS

No Meat Erections

The best thing you can do to keep you and your penis in good shape and functioning properly (besides exercise and laying off booze and cigarettes) is to give your body a healthy, low-cholesterol, balanced diet.

High cholesterol can coat and block arteries and veins and reduce the blood flow to your testicles and penis, let alone your heart and head. Every time you consume more cholesterol, it increases the risk of not being able to have an erection. Some reports estimate that for every point of increase in one's total cholesterol, the risk of erection dysfunction increases 1.5 times.

Maybe that saying, "Real men don't eat quiche," isn't so bogus after all. Perhaps folks who don't eat any dairy or animal products (Vegans) are on to something good. It sounds like men with low cholesterol diets are more likely to get erections when desired than those who chow down on meat, eggs and potatoes.

If Your Penis Could Talk

Duck Therapy

When the guy I'm attached to was six years old, his father would take us down to the local YMCA for a swim. They had a public pool with different hours for men and women. Nobody wore swimsuits. We all just ran around in what we were born with.

One day, as we were coming out of the pool, my boy realized that for some reason I had gotten hard and was sticking out like a sore thumb. He just stood there staring at me, wondering what I was doing. His older brother came up to us and said, "Control yourself!"

My prominence must have caught the lifeguard's attention, because before I knew it he was grabbing my boy's hand and making him walk awkwardly around the pool. He told us, "Just walk like this and it will go away." He put his feet out and waddled like a duck. The kid I'm attached to was about to laugh, but realized the lifeguard was totally serious.

He gave it a try, without quacking, and saw that the lifeguard must have had a lot of experience with this kind of thing. Within minutes I was my regular flaccid self, flapping between his legs like a worm looking for a place to dig. I've had a strange connection with pools and ducks ever since.

PENIS FACTS

Early to Bed, Early to Rise

The majority of erections during sleep happen in the early hours of the morning because that is when testosterone levels in the blood are at their highest level. That period is called *Nocturnal Penile Tumescence (NPT).* NPT takes place from birth to advanced old age. It typically happens in three episodes a night for a total of two to three hours. Scientists measure NPT by placing the penis inside an expandable ring.

If our partners could harness this nightly activity for their personal pleasure, without waking us up, we would open our eyes in the morning to saturated and exhausted lovers!

5

Up, Up and Away

If you were telling a woman, or someone who has never experienced sex, what it feels like to have an erection and orgasm, what would you say?

Author's note: *Though the terminology varied, the sensations, emotions, feelings and physical reactions men shared regarding erections and orgasm were substantively and fundamentally identical. It seems that we have all gone to the same school and learned the same language but have different accents, histories and interpretations.*

An erection feels like a gathering of attention, of everything being concentrated in a pleasurable way. The body relaxes and this involuntary thing happens. When I was a teenager I would get erections when I didn't want to, which was frightening. I couldn't control it. The sensation itself, though, is a kind of centering. Something growing and becoming more and more sensitive.

To me, it's almost painful. Pleasure is only a part of it. It's painful pleasure. It's a focusing and gathering, as though the rest of my body is draining. I need to bring attention to it. If my wanger is just standing there all by itself it hurts, but when it receives attention pleasure occurs. The whole process builds and builds and builds until it's unbearable, with all the condensing of juices. Then when I have an orgasm it's a complete release. There's also the wreath of emotions surrounding us, that has a great deal to do with how much pleasure we experience. I've always believed that it's important to satisfy the woman, and that affects my pleasure.

It's a two-pronged event—giving pleasure and receiving pleasure. The more I give the more I receive. It took me awhile to understand that. When I was young and just concentrated on myself it seemed like something was missing.

It's like water building up behind the dam, with pressure that needs to be released. Maybe it's psychological, because it tends to happen like that only when another person is involved.

When I first become aware that an erection is coming on, I have the sense that I'm in a crowded room and my penis is another person. I see my penis and we wink at each other. We have this inside joke, and we say, "Yeah." That's the beginning of the hard-on for me, that first recognition and sense of pending release and ecstasy of the orgasm. Preferably an orgasm is a moment of shared ecstasy—a confluence of two excited human beings. There's nothing like that.

It's like a gift you're giving each other, giving and receiving.

The downside of orgasm is the ephemeralness of the actual orgasm. It's so fucking short. A woman's just stays up there and ours is just up and down. The post-orgasm state is so quick.

Though it feels awkward to have something firm protruding from your body where it normally doesn't, an erection creates an intense need for the penis to be touched. It's difficult to leave it alone when it's erect. It's even better when somebody else touches it. There are different kinds of erections. There's the kind when you wake up in the morning needing to pee and have to wait until your cock goes down. That's what I call a functional erection—your body doing something without your being aware. It doesn't even feel that great. Then there's the conspicuous erection, which I first became aware of while watching TV with my parents. Something arousing would come on and I'd have to hide my erection from my parents. And then there's the kind of erection that's just right, when you're about to have sex, when you can embrace the feeling and enjoy the firmness. There's a shift in your perceptions, you become focused on the end result—getting off. You tend to lose sight of other things in your life, the little things, duties, aches and pains. Your whole focus shifts to ending the erection with an orgasm.

When I'm with someone and have a really powerful orgasm it's different than when I'm on my own. I can feel the semen coming out. It feels like a whole body thing. It's not restricted to my groin. It emanates. It's like jumping off a high place, a plateau. You're up really high, nervous and scared about falling off. Then you just jump off and don't care if you land or fly. You can feel the wind rushing past and see the view and you just float in that beautiful space. There's no thought, just pure sensation. I'm compulsive about a lot of things, including sex. I like the ritual, because thought is absent for a while and I'm not so bound up in my crazy life.

An erection takes my head to the head of my penis. All my thoughts are there. I'm thinking about how good it feels. It feels exciting. It's a coalescing of everything in one spot. It's all the emotions. There's about a ten-second squeeze above my right testicle, which is followed by feeling the semen flowing through my body and shooting out. I can have a second orgasm with oral sex rather quickly, but it is usually less intense and distinctive.

Having an erection is like being on a precipice, on an edge. You either step back and clear your head or fall off and find out what it's like on the other side. When you orgasm, you can't do anything about it; there's nothing to control or grab onto. If you get experienced at it, you surrender to what's on the other side.

An erection causes a sense of tightness, which puts more density out at the end. I can feel the entire curve of my penis coming out of my tailbone—a sense of weight and bounce that comes back up the shaft. My skin becomes hypersensitive. Heading into orgasm, either through masturbation or with another person, I feel like my brain goes away and all my consciousness and awareness goes down into my penis. I become a gigantic urge to thrust. Then I'm working towards a threshold. It feels like something is about to happen. When I get there I feel like I've entered the Schwarzchilde Radius. Outside is the normal world but inside that radius everything is sucked into one place. This electrical charge comes up, with a rushing sense of energy, and nothing will stop it. I can feel the pulses in my penis, like a pleasurable burst of energy exploding in the base of my brain. With each pump comes incredible pleasure. When it's over I feel like a wet rag lying limp on my partner.

An erection feels like a fifteen-minute sneeze. It starts by feeling really warm and exciting throughout my whole body, with a focus in my groin. An orgasm feels like the top blowing off of everything.

An erection brings everything into the present and makes the rest of the body feel more involved than at other times. An orgasm feels like a powerful release of energy.

An orgasm is contained euphoria. You're flying, like in a flipped-out drug thing. Bliss, happiness. When you're with a woman, you can feel the give and take and experience a oneness with the other person. It feels a lot better with someone else, than by yourself.

When I was in my first year of high school and was near a girl I would often get an erection that wouldn't go down. It would stay that way for an uncomfortably long period of time, making it difficult to sit. I did a lot of standing in those days.

An erection makes me feel like a part of my body has a life of it's own. The funny thing is that when I touch it, it feels like it's separate and connected at the same time. I'm holding something in my hand that feels ten times bigger and warmer, yet it's still me. It feels like it's connected to me at the groin and going back into my gut. One of the wonderful things is that some parts of my penis are more sensitive than others. I tell my partner it can be like a quick trip down to the park or a long journey that you want to go on and on.

It's like an erupting volcano. More and more pressure builds up until it has to release out the top. It's the ultimate sensual experience. It's like when you have a really bad itch from poison oak and scratch it. The sensation you get is so overwhelming that you can't think of any externals, because it itches so bad and scratching feels so good.

An orgasm is warm, comfortable and absolutely safe. It is being completely open, unafraid of anything and naked in a total sense. It was wonderful discovering that. It's like a river that has risen far too high. There's so much water going by it has to spill over the banks and flood. It also feels like a pleasurable electric shock through my whole torso. It can reach up to the top of my head. Physically, it is the greatest pleasure I've every known. When I first made love with women I found that there was much I hadn't learned from knowing my own body. But knowing my own body first helped me to fully enjoy sex with another. Someone once said, "To masturbate is sweet and to fuck is divine."

An orgasm feels like a strange, funny tingling feeling taking over most of my body in a nice, powerful, complete and wonderful way.

Prior to the erection it feels like a lava bed being stirred. It has both sympathetic and emotional components, and has to be shared with an individual who is capable of emotional vulnerability as well as clear expression. Someone who is really conscious of what they are saying. There has to be some subterranean aliveness.

It feels like a swelling, a heightening, an opening of awareness and a sharpening or pointedness. Each orgasm is individual; it's hard to categorize. It's situational. It can feel like a rush of expansion.

The first time I ejaculated I was surprised. I didn't know what I was experiencing. It felt like a visitor from another planet. There was no context. I had received no instruction or education from my father and I was the only male in the household besides him. And as a teenager I was pretty isolated. It was the early 1970s and I think our school had been left out of the "sexual revolution."

It sort of feels like embracing the heavens. It's very uplifting. It also involves feelings of vulnerability, openness and excitement. There's a sense of being exposed, naked—no posturing or hiding behind anything. An orgasm feels like leaving one's body, like being consumed in love. To me there are different kinds of orgasms. Love takes it to a depth and height that is spiritual. It touches all one's senses. With masturbation it's more like a primordial physicality.

An orgasm is like a building up of energy and then a release that feels ecstatic. It feels like fingers of electricity all over you.

An erection feels like all this energy coming together in one part of your body. It makes you feel intensely alive.

Having an orgasm—at least a good one—feels like a whole body-consciousness experience. It feels like my entire spine and the top of my head are released. That kind of orgasm, an out-of-body experience, is rare. Sex by myself feels more like a release of energy, of sexual tension.

If Your Penis Could Talk

The Wedding

We were so excited. Tyler had been in love before, or at least thought he had. But when we... I mean me, his penis, and the rest of him met Juanita, we found out what real love was all about.

After about a year and a half of going out and getting to know one another (her vagina and I became best friends), we ... he ... they decided to get married.

It was a real big bash. All their relatives, friends, even some old lovers were there to wish them well and celebrate their life together. They had a big traditional church wedding, which her Mexican-Catholic family really appreciated. Afterwards they had a feast, dance and reception at the parish hall that went on late into the evening.

Tyler and Juanita drank and talked and danced along with everyone else, and enjoyed the love and attention. I found myself getting a little woozy. At around two in the morning we climbed into our car and were driven to the luxury hotel that had been booked for our honeymoon night.

After they had put away their bags, taken off their tuxedo, wedding dress and under-clothes, they eyed each other, and me and my friend, passionately. They fell into bed kissing, stroking and laughing.

I could feel Tyler's excitement, in fact I could feel both their excitement, but realized I wasn't moving. No matter what they did or tried to do to me, I just lay there.

I heard him say, "I'm so drunk."

She answered, "Me too."

They both started laughing again and wrestling and tickling each other until we all fell off the bed.

Somehow they managed to get us back in bed and it wasn't long until they were both snoring away.

In the morning, before Tyler woke up, I could feel Juanita's hand, then her mouth waking me up. She slowly left me and kissed her way up to Tyler's face. He opened his eyes and smiled. He could feel me hard as a tree in her hand and it wasn't long until we were all fucking madly away.

The wedding night hadn't finished the way they had expected it to, but the morning after was ten times better.

We've all been enjoying each other's company for about five years now and keep learning new ways to give each other pleasure and love. They have their disagreements and misunderstandings, but it seems like Juanita's vagina and I are going to be seeing each other for a long time to come.

PENIS FACTS

Stuck Like Glue

A lot of people have heard stories about dogs getting stuck together while mating and all kinds of things being done to free them. Whether they actually get stuck, or the purveyors of such stories merely feel uncomfortable witnessing dogs mating, is uncertain.

This got me to wondering if people have ever become mired while copulating, or if getting stuck is even possible. I'd heard folks joke about couples having to call 911 to get unentwined, but had never actually seen evidence that these accounts were true.

It turns out that the subject has been taken seriously. The *British Medical Journal* once published a story from a doctor who claimed to have seen a couple come into the emergency room *penile captivus* (penis stuck in the vagina). However, no such incidents have ever been substantiated. Even if the head of a man's penis were to become greatly swollen in size and width during intercourse, the vagina has no way to permanently capture it or hold it inside. Although, if one were going to be captured I can't think of a nicer place to be held prisoner.

If Your Penis Could Talk

Almost Fatal Attraction

My man and I have never been as openly wanted or desired as we were when he was in a writing class at the university. A pretty tight group of people attended this class for about ten weeks every year. One summer we even continued the class after it was officially over, meeting in people's homes. Even the professor joined the home group.

There was a girl in this class who was engaged, until she told us that the engagement had been broken off in a very bad way. During the next class, after she had made that announcement, she started talking to Ben, the man I'm attached to. He was feeling sick that day and left early, but she followed us and told him they should get together for dinner sometime.

He said that would be fine, someday. She kept following him to the car and said, "...so we could talk."

He said, "Sure, we can talk about anything you like."

She said, "How about we talk about wild sex?"

He ignored her remark, got in the car and left.

The next day, when we were walking back to class, this same woman walked up, grabbed Ben's hand and started walking with us. Ben felt weird. He didn't know what she was doing.

After class, while Ben was talking with a friend, the lady interrupted the conversation and wrapped her body around us. Ben said, "Hey girl, get off of me."

The next week things went from weird to weirder. The professor wanted two people to do a dialogue in front of the class. This woman picked Ben. We went up, did the dialogue, then sat down and everyone in class wrote about it. At the end of the class she walked by and dropped what she'd written on Ben's desk before following some friends into the hallway. He opened her paper. I could feel a twinge surge through me. It must have been a pretty hot letter.

As we walked out of the class she said loudly to Ben, right in front of a group of students, "I wonder if you're good in bed?"

He said, "I don't know. I think we'd have to practice. What are you doing on Friday night?"

She said she was busy on Friday, but Saturday would be great.

I don't think Ben really wanted to go, but since she'd said it in public he felt he had to act cool and macho. As far as I knew, and I would be the one to know, he had never had a one-night stand and wasn't really very attracted to this girl. She was pretty, but the chemistry wasn't there.

True to his word, however, Ben went over to her house on Saturday night, toothbrush in tow.

When we arrived it all felt real awkward and forced. She kept giving Ben drinks and said, "Here, this will help." They both got plastered.

Finally, she said, "Are you going to kiss me?"

With that invitation he went for it. They ended up clumsily pulling each other's clothes off and falling into bed. They did a lot of kissing, fondling and stroking, but Ben was so drunk he couldn't send me the blood I needed to rise. I could tell he felt real bad about it and was embarrassed.

The next morning she almost kicked us out of bed and told Ben to get lost. It was then that he realized he had simply been used to try to get some kind of revenge on her ex-fiancée.

Ben was feeling dirty and like a sexual failure. It was apparent that she had no feelings for him. She never showed up for another writing class after that, but Ben was so furious that he tracked her down and told her on the phone how she had made him feel. I think I could even hear her crying on the other end.

We never heard from her again, and Ben has never had a woman so brazenly come on to him (and me) since.

PENIS FACTS

"Did You Come?" "Yes, Did You?"

Male and female genitals come from the same fetal tissue.

Despite the anatomical differences between male and female genitals, and the assumption that we experience sex differently, it turns out that orgasms in men and women are physiologically and psychologically very similar. Studies have been done in which experts could not reliably determine gender when reading descriptions of orgasms with all anatomical references removed.

Researchers have also discovered that multi-orgasmic men (repeated orgasm without ejaculation) have the same arousal charts in the laboratory as multi-orgasmic women.

The next time you think a woman doesn't understand what you're saying, thinking or feeling (because she's a woman), think again!

6

Sing Along with Dick

If your penis could carry a tune, what song would it sing?

Jumping Jack Flash
When the Red Red Robin Comes Bob-Bob-Bobbin' Along
I'm in the Mood for Love
Hey, Hey, Up She's Rising Early in the Morning
Higher Ground
What Should We Do with a Drunken Sailor?
I Gotta Be Me
Please Release Me, Let Me Go
The Theme Song to Shaft.
You Can't Always Get What You Want
All of Me
Coming Through the Rhine
When I'm Sixty-Four

I've Been Everywhere, Man
O Solo Mia
Hallelujah
I've Been Working on the Railroad
A Secret Love
Walking on Sunshine
Oh Happy Day
Downtown
Dreamweaver
You Can't Always Get What You Want
Happy Birthday
Swing Low Sweet Chariot
Balls of Fire
Honeysuckle Rose
Lean on Me
Amazing Grace
Zippity Do Da, Zippity A
Born To Be Wild
Twist and Shout
Coming Round the Mountain When She Comes
Crazy
You've Got a Friend
Wild Horses
Fever
I'm So Excited
Honey Pie
Jigging It
I've Got Rhythm
Trouble
Superstition

If Your Penis Could Talk

The End of an Era

Recently, a sharp, thin blunt object was forced into my testicle buddies and the main switches to my reproductive energy were permanently disconnected. I found it ironic that this procedure was performed. After all, I had done my job so well. We'd had three children in a row. Now the route to the semen was cut off at the pass. I wouldn't be able to produce another kid.

At first I wondered if I'd ever be the same. Would I still be able to get it up? Was my man still a man? What would men in other cultures think of this?

It actually turned out pretty cool. We didn't have to worry about birth control anymore and could just let the good times roll!

Three's a Crowd

I wasn't always the smartest guy around, but I sure had fun when we were younger. We enjoyed women of all types and personalities, though few relationships lasted for very long. Almost anything that moved and would let us in was a thrill.

I remember a trip I made to Europe once, where I met a couple who wanted me to join them in some sexual play. I'd never been with two people at once. I must say it was a surprising treat to be touched and sucked and fucked by both the man and the woman. We'd all do it together, then each person would receive all the attention of the other two. After awhile I didn't know which way was up.

The only painful experience was once when I was ready to enter a vagina and the woman who owned it said, "No." That was a bummer. I'd been on the verge of exploding for about an hour when she changed her mind. I could have lived with that. After all it was her body. But it was as frustrating as having someone hold my favorite dish before my eyes and then, just as I was about to take a bite, put a clear plastic cover over it. I could see the food, but I couldn't taste it!

PENIS FACTS

Again and Again and Again

Men can have multiple orgasms without ejaculating. You heard me right—*multiple* orgasms *without* ejaculating. Though they seem to occur simultaneously, an orgasm takes place seconds before ejaculation. If you learn to stop, control and/or delay coming, you can have an orgasm, retain your erection and come again and again. It takes practice and concentrated awareness of your body, but you can't go wrong because you end up having an orgasm either way, and you can practice alone or with your partner.

Without ejaculation, the semen is reabsorbed into the body and the orgasmic contractions massage the prostate, which actually enhances health and vitality. You get all the pleasure combined with the added benefit of knowing it's good for your health, too! Sort of like a tasty low-fat meal.

There are a number of books that talk about this Chinese Taoist technique and philosophy called *Sexual Kung Fu*. I would highly recommend *The Multi-Orgasmic Man: How Any Man Can Experience Multiple Orgasm and Dramatically Enhance His Sexual Relationship*. Its authors are Mantak Chia and Douglas Abrams.

If Your Penis Could Talk

What Might Have Been

My man was with one woman for quite some time. Finally he was forced to take her behavior at face value and accept the fact that it was over.

He began to get interested in someone else, and she seemed attracted to him, but it was a delicate situation because they were close neighbors. My man and her children were friends. They decided it would be better not to get involved sexually (which always affects me deeply).

More time passed and they talked about it again. The next thing you know I was taking the lead and she was responding. Then my man needed to leave town for a couple of weeks. He left a note asking to see her when he returned, and expressing great anticipation. During the course of the trip he decided to disregard the consequences and go for it when he got back.

But, as usual, it wasn't so simple. During the trip he spoke with his ex-partner and there was a note of sweetness and reconciliation in her voice. He'd always found her incredibly erotic and, having been with her for some time, was swayed by the conversation.

When he returned from his trip the first person he encountered was his ex-partner. They had a wonderful reunion and an exquisite peak experience. At the same time, he realized there was this other person he'd left weeks earlier who was waiting for his return as well.

He decided he should contact her and tell her that he couldn't see her anymore because he was back with his ex. But when he met his neighbor, common sense failed to overcome my powers. Though they stopped short of completing the act, they got pretty heated up. Reason eventually prevailed, though, and he didn't go through with it. He told her about his ex and they parted.

Almost simultaneously, his ex found out about his new lover and decided that was too much of an affront for her to handle, so she wouldn't have anything to do with him either. The end result was that once again my man and I were left to fend for ourselves.

7

Dic-tating or Dic-tation

How much does your penis and sex influence who you are, how you see yourself and how you relate to women and men?

Author's note: *This dialogue deeply touched the hearts of the men interviewed, and made us question how much of our behavior is biological—imbedded in our chromosomes—and how much is learned—absorbed from our surroundings and culture. I believe that, in some respects, it doesn't matter. The real question is not where our behavior comes from, but whether we can see ourselves honestly, enjoy the drives, urges and differences that we live with, and make responsible decisions and choices that respect and honor other human beings.*

Whenever I'm talking to a woman I'm aware of a sexual dimension. There are probably times it doesn't happen, but usually it does. It seems like there's always a sexual field, like gravity. I'm always calling roll, checking out the women I'm attracted to. I monitor my behavior, but I'm aware of what's going on. Some men have lost their jobs because they didn't pay attention and let their dick rule.

This probably isn't cool to say, but the first things I look at when I see or meet a woman are her breasts. I try to look at her eyes and the rest of body, but her breasts are the first visible sign to me that she's a woman and they stick right out there, almost at eye level.

I know that I sexually monitor women, but I also check out men as sexual beings, mostly as competition, but occasionally as sexual partners as well. Sometimes I'm not aware of these feelings at all, while at other times I am. I don't know where they come from. They just seem natural and affect every relationship I have in some way.

There's a line in a Toni Morrison novel where a main character, a woman, is walking downtown and all the old men are talking. The line reads, "The old men's lust has turned to kindness." Sometimes I disguise my lust with kindness. I don't do that with men, but I do with women.

I recently became aware of an analytical tool called SWOT Analysis, which stands for Strengths, Weaknesses, Opportunity and Threat. It feels sort of primal. When I meet a guy, I check him out as a threat—he could steal a girl I want. With a woman I realize I'm checking out her strengths and the opportunity. I do that with everybody I meet. Because I'm heterosexual, there's more of a sexual component with a woman then with a man. At work, I'm currently the boss of three women. I'm aware of myself thinking about them as potential sexual conquests. Then I just tell myself, "No, I can't go there. I can't do that." I have to be totally aboveboard and fair with these people—even more so than if they were men.

I objectify and evaluate and constantly wonder what this or that woman would be like. It gives me a sense of power, though I don't actually have any. It's like a "monkey mind" and that's all that it is. It doesn't have to affect my behavior and I realize sometimes how disconnected it is from others. I wonder, "What would they be like?" I used to feel guilty about it, but now I realize it's a reflex and let it go.

I was fortunate to work in an office with three women and four men. We talked all day about sex. We would do our work, but someone would start a conversation and off we'd go. You couldn't do that nowadays. That was when I realized that women think of sex, too.

My sexuality is a huge part of who I am. I don't feel like I'm totally driven by my cock, or that my sexuality is detrimental to my life and relationships, but at the same time I think its subtle influence colors everything I do and every interaction I have with people. When I don't see myself as being sexually attractive, or viable, my self-image suffers dramatically. If I don't see myself in a positive sexual way, then I don't see myself positively in other ways either. Luckily, most of the time, I do feel good about my sexuality.

Working in construction, I wondered for a long time if the other guys questioned my sexual orientation, because I have an accent, and a vocabulary, and appear to be intelligent. For a while I felt compelled to overemphasize my sexuality by talking about women a lot, and by commenting on women who walked by the job site. It wasn't because I was really interested in the women walking by, or in sharing my sexual exploits, but I felt I had to prove my heterosexuality. With women, I always have in the back of my mind that this is a possible sexual partner and I need to project a certain confidence, humor, coolness and likeability to make a sexual encounter possible. It's difficult to have sexual feelings and not get caught up in the expectation of having it happen.

On some unconscious level, my penis decides what I'm looking at or what I want to look at. I'm not sure how it works, but if I'm driving along somewhere and I see a woman, I'll look longer than a casual glance. That's when I think my sexuality and my maleness decide what I'm going to linger on. Even if I see a couple of women from behind, when I get in front of them my eyes go to my mirror to see their front.

I find that my sexual desire has made me embarrassed and shy around women, because I think about them sexually and don't want them to know it. When I used to go pick up my wife at work, I had to walk through all the women working there and it made me real uncomfortable.

I'm not embarrassed to be naked in front of women. I rather enjoy it. There was the free love revolution, and then there was a time in the seventies when you had to be really cautious, because sex could mean a commitment. Sometimes I would want to be mentally committed before I got physically committed. The older I am, the more relaxed I am with my feminine side. I welcome its emergence. I see it as having compassion. It's *not* thinking with my dick. It's kind of like becoming asexual and being more centered in my heart.

I'm heterosexual and married and grateful to have a like-minded person to share my sex with. But we are also together because of our heart connection and spiritual oneness. We are on the same spiritual path. Sex is the icing on the cake, whereas in the past it *was* the cake. At this time in my life there is no way I would ever have sex with someone besides my wife. I approach women as sisters and men as brothers. And since I don't want to have sex with my sister, sex is no longer part of the equation with other women. It doesn't even come up. Because of that I have a lot of female friends.

On a scale from one to ten, sex is ten. My penis rules. I can't think of any other factor that supercedes that consideration—my sexuality, my tingle meter. My surroundings are work, family (home) and the public sphere. The most difficult of those for me is work. If there is someone I want to have sex with at work, how can I do it without jeopardizing my career? The price that I pay for not following my desires at work is a nervous tension that I have to release in other ways. An attractive female body is one thing, but a beautiful body combined with intelligence takes it over the top for me. I have to engage in a lot of self-talk about what I'm doing and check in with and gauge my tingle-meter. One side of my brain is talking intellectual stuff while the other side is checking out my physical reactions. I ask myself how far away I am from the person, what messages I'm giving her.

If I lament one thing about my sexuality it is that I'm predictable. It seems like Madison Avenue figured me out and I've never been able to get away from the idea that I want a woman I have sex with to look a certain way. If she doesn't look that way I'm not aroused. As a result there have been some women who were overweight that I found attractive, but when I had the opportunity to be sexual with them I felt short-changed during the interaction. I asked myself, "Why am I with her?" The way a woman looks has something to do with my worth, with how I think others see me. Even the woman I'm married to needs to fit a certain image. I don't like that about myself, but I don't know what to do about it.

I am always conscious, when I meet a woman, of evaluating her as an object. It's like targeting software. The software does the evaluation automatically. I am conscious of that and say, "Down boy." I am always aware of the possibility of having sex with that woman. It is a constant chatter in my mind. If I've got the time, and I'm in a meeting or something, I'll indulge in a fantasy and wonder what she would be like. If I'm involved in a task that needs to get done, I just put it in the rubbish bin and think about it later. I don't think women are aware of what I'm doing. I've become very good at masking those feelings, especially in professional situations. I've been very careful to not project those feelings. My outside behavior appears proper, even though inside I may be having all these reactions. I never want my reactions to be someone else's problem. I also recognize that it's my targeting system and my genetics, not theirs. I hold the worldview that men want to spread their seed, for genetics, and women don't. I accept the feelings, but don't act on them.

I always felt a really strong connection to my sexuality. I used to let it control me. Although I still feel very much affected by it, I've been able to acknowledge and appreciate it without letting it control my decisions. I've tried hard to do that without stifling my sexuality. It's like being able to look and appreciate without touching. I get joy from observing. Whenever you try to squelch any emotion it doesn't work and usually creates the opposite. I try to acknowledge what's there.

There have been times in my life when my relationships with women on a business level have been clearly impacted by my sexual attraction to them—by my efforts to bed them down. There have been times when I have purposefully encouraged a relationship—one that started as a business relationship—because of my sexual interest. I've used my maleness as a power thing. Throughout much of my life I've maintained an authoritative, righteous perspective on things, which I attribute in large measure to my father. I have manipulated circumstances and relationships to sexually entice women.

Sometimes I've wanted to achieve fame in order to attract women. To my knowledge, I have never gotten in trouble because of it. Politics and power can be very sexually stimulating, which is quite clear from the public perspective. It seems less of an issue for me now that I'm partnered and older. When I was single and younger, and in that game, it was much more important. So, as long as I'm hooked up, I rarely think about being with someone else. In the old days, I thought about it often and developed strategies to see if I could make it with so-and-so.

When I was working I had more women friends than men friends. They were always more touchy, and I wondered if they were coming on to me, or if it was just how they were. If I wanted to maintain a strictly working relationship, I would kid around with these women and then go back to work. If I wanted to get in some girl's knickers I'd be on my best behavior and we'd get together outside of the office.

We're bound to what we are. I am very aware of myself as a male. I am not just this body. How I live with my body is also part of who I am. Furthermore, how I live with myself has everything to do with how I live with others. At this time in my life, I am conscious of my body. When I feel healthy I feel close to my entire body, my sexuality and my penis. When I don't feel well, it's the opposite. I think about all adults—both male and female—in sexual terms. I see them as partners with others. Men have penises, women have vaginas and as long as we continue having these parts, we'll be around.

I don't love men the same way I love women. I'm not attracted to men, nor do I usually want to spend much time with them. Women tend to be more interesting to me. Most men are unable to talk about real things in the world, at least in the American culture. It is not the same in all cultures. Not many men attract me, but women usually do. I have a full relationship with my woman partner, whom I love. Having a full and growing relationship with my partner takes the two of us to a lovemaking place that is solely ours, that nobody else can experience.

I have a lot of empathy for men who think women are different from them, are afraid of that difference, and believe that the only way to approach women is from a place of power or control. When a man recognizes and validates that belief system, he can usually acknowledge and let go of the vulnerability and fear that produce it. I saw this clearly when a relationship I was in fell apart. Losing this woman made me aware that I was viewing her largely through many of my own assumptions and images.

Men don't usually come into contact with women in non-sexually predicated ways, either in groups or individually, so we tend to respond to women with culturally reinforced conditioning. Having a chance to pursue relationships that don't fit this paradigm is fabulously enriching. Though gender differences exist, we don't have to focus on them. We can learn to let go of a lot of the junk we've been taught about love, sex, and women, and choose to be with them without hiding our fear behind a wall of control or manipulation.

I'm penis driven and it's gotten me into trouble. It makes me feel one-sided. I wish I could be more balanced. On the other hand, sexuality is extremely important to me and I don't want to discount that aspect of my life. I take turns reconciling these opposites. I try to recognize what's going on in a given situation and decide what to do—to have some perspective on it.

When I was celibate, my attitude towards women was different. Scoring was clearly not an objective at that time. And, because I was not athletic or aggressive, it was just as difficult for me to be close to boys as girls. Boys were too physically aggressive for me. That changed some when I became a Brother. I had no sexual desire during that time. Once I left the order and began having relationships with women, I found it a lot easier to communicate with women than with men, in both nonsexual and sexual ways. I think that is because I regard women as more sensitive and interested in people, emotions and spirituality. I'm also a pacifist, so beating up other guys and going to war are things I never wanted to do. Stereotypical adolescent male behavior was something I never identified with or experienced. My father was much the same way. He never said it, but I picked it up nonverbally. I am the fifth generation in my family to not marry until after the age of forty. That fact has made me wonder what material we are made of, and to what degree postponing sexual experience represents genetic bias.

The comedian/actor Robin Williams once said, "God gave us all a penis and a brain, but only enough blood to run one at a time."

My sexuality is definitely a big part of who I am, and my relationships with women are part of my sexuality. I have many lady friends that I feel sexual towards, but don't necessarily have sex with. The sexuality is manifested with them in different ways, such as dialogue and being with them in a way that does not involve my masculinity. I talk with them about things that I don't normally talk about with men.

When I was younger I was a womanizer and, as the expression goes, followed my dick. But after years of letting it lead me around I felt extremely empty, unhappy and unfulfilled. I was spiritually bankrupt and didn't like what I saw in myself, so I set out to find an answer. One day a friend of mine, who was traveling on his way to Japan, loaned me a book called *The Diamond Sutra*. After he left I started reading it. It opened up doors and made me stop, look, listen, see and feel in ways that I had not up until that time. It introduced me to silence and created a desire for inner silence.

I used to do a lot of consulting for companies where I had to come up with ideas and concepts. I was hired once by a group to come up with concepts in three days. It turned out that the entire group was composed of women, except for myself. It was exhilarating, because when they approached the subject it was so different than what I was used to as a male. It was profoundly organic, unstructured and open. I was dumbfounded at how they related and worked together. The creativity was astounding. I felt sort of out of place, like a dick. My thought process was so structured and straight-line.

The experience helped me to realize more clearly how I saw myself in the world. It made me realize that, as a male, my universe was narrow, in the sense that, I was "the doer," whereas the environment with the women was more like "being" and "receiving." For example, if a group of men got on a sailboat, they would decide who was going to do what, who would be the Captain and plot a course. My sense is that if it were a group of women, they would find consensus over who would have which role and be more open to their course and to changes in their destination.

I'd say my cock is in charge about 10 to 15 percent of the time, and occasionally I have to remind myself that I'm in a committed relationship. As I've gotten older I've become more aware of the energy I'm sending out, and what I'm receiving. I intentionally try not to send out sexual vibes with women. When they come on to me, I resist by ignoring it and not feeding energy into it. What has made the difference for me is having a partner who is very aware of this issue, and who points out to me when I am acting in a sexually predatory way. I've started to become personally responsible for the messages I am sending out to people and it has been very healing. I used to confuse sex with care and love.

I used to follow my urges and sexual attractions instead of my head. Now I set aside time for sex and keep more control over it. I try to know people better before I consider becoming sexually involved. Sometimes I let the sexual aspect go altogether and just have a friendship. It was OK when I followed my penis around, and it was good to discover how to use it in new ways, but there's also a time to learn how to control it. You can hurt others and yourself when you base a relationship totally on sex.

PENIS FACTS

What Every Penis Should Know.

When the pubucoccygeal (PC) muscle is strengthened it can provide strong erections, more control over ejaculation and intense orgasms. When you tighten your muscles to stop the flow while urinating, you are working the PC muscle. It is very similar to the kegel muscle in women. You can strengthen this muscle by squeezing and releasing it, doing 50 repititions several times throughout the day. You can literally be exercising your cock in public and nobody will know.

If Your Penis Could Talk

Love the One You're With

I'm a searcher. I expect there are many like me. What has dogged me in my adult years is restlessness . . . the search. There's a reason the man to whom I'm attached is on his third marriage. I think it's because he is trying to find a way to confirm, confront, or deal with my restlessness.

When he got married the first time, I was in denial of my need to be non-exclusive, not to fit in just one pocket. I wanted to experience a variety of joys and curiosities. In that first marriage I created a great deal of hurt because of my searching and restlessness. He was unable to articulate my needs to his spouse so we cheated in search of pleasure with others.

In his second marriage he was more aware of his responsibility to state my needs, but the awareness was still new and he didn't express himself well. He brought a third party into the marriage, creating a sexual triad, but that didn't seem to help.

Entering into his third marriage, at forty-one, he didn't feel like beating around the bush. When he first met his third wife he told her right away that he was not sexually exclusive, but that he wanted an intimate, committed relationship. She agreed and said that would work for her as well.

Our days of being in the shadows about our sexuality are now over, which has brought a great deal of relief. Of course, the new challenge is, if he is not going to be exclusive, neither is she. In fact, her experiences have benefited me. She is bisexual, and every now and then she meets a woman who is searching in her life and my man and I get to be part of their love relationship.

It's all been about finding a balance in our sexuality and his desire to have a family. My man doesn't understand why people, if they are honest with themselves, can't have both. It's not as though God sends down your mate from heaven above. The person you're likely to meet is usually close by, even right next door.

8

Sunshine and Shadows

What's the best thing your penis has ever done? What's the worst?

Author's note: *This was not an easy question. When asked in groups, few men revealed anything they (or their penis) had ever done that was wrong, or felt like it was wrong. On the other hand, they were eager to share the best thing their penis had done. Yet, when we were away from the earshot of others, many men told me about things they had done in their younger years for which they still felt ashamed—things they had not told anyone before. Describing those incidents doesn't change the past or insinuate that the men should be forgiven for what they did. But it is heartening to know that these men have taken responsibility for their behavior and not blamed the person they took advantage of.*

There have been times in my life when I was totally driven by sexual desire. I went out on a double date in high school with a girl named Julie. She was a sweet girl. I was all over her, reaching under her skirt. She was terrified. She was trying so hard to be nice. Later I felt ashamed of my behavior. I remember other times like that when I felt driven in a mindless sort of way. To me, that was the worst. Completely disregarding the other human being because I was so intent on getting off.

The best, absolutely divine times were those moments of sexual bliss with a woman that were ultimate, satisfying and transcendent. All restraints fell away and it felt like I was soaring through the cosmos. I can reduce those moments to a few. Sometimes we think such moments are occurring with our partner when they're not, but there have been times when I knew the bliss was shared, and those were the best moments I've experienced in my life. The ecstasy transcends feeling. If there is nirvana, that's it. My ego vanishes.

For me the best and worst experiences were the same incidents. The worst thing was when I was younger and attempting to have intercourse and losing my erection. After I had experienced this on different occasions I realized that it was a signal that I wasn't comfortable being with that particular person. So, in another way it was the best thing, since it taught me something important about intimacy and finding the right match. After that everything changed.

The worst thing my penis has ever been through happened when I was looking for some kind of lubricant with which to pleasure myself and chose dandruff shampoo. Whatever is in that stuff was awful. It ended up causing the skin on the end of my penis to peel off. It was terribly painful.

The best thing my penis did was to help end my relationship with my first wife. I had fallen in love with the woman who became my second wife, while still married to the first. The person I was married to and I were even trying to get pregnant. One night we were in the middle of having sex and I realized, "Oh my God, what am I doing?" I took the opportunity to discuss my fears and to explain that I didn't want to have children. That confession opened the door out of the relationship and marked the beginning of one that has worked much better.

The best thing my penis has done is to serve as a conduit to discharge all the urine I've created in my life. If it hadn't done it's job so well, I'd be one big, bloated, toxic mess by now.

The worst was not being able to control my ejaculations. It seems that as soon as my penis gets close to a vagina, I ejaculate. It's something I've always been embarrassed about—not having more control. Thank goodness it only happens in private, when we are both naked and not when I have my clothes on, otherwise I'd be creaming my pants every time a woman and her vagina passed by.

I had sex once with my girlfriend and she was so drunk she didn't know it. She was almost unconscious. Since then, I've had a residual feeling of guilt because I didn't really have her consent. I never got the chance to apologize because I haven't seen her for twelve years and have no idea where she is now.

Being with two women at once was definitely my best experience. Having two partners compounded the emotional and physical intensity of the sex and made it twice as sensual. There was a lot of attachment and letting go of that attachment and embracing both at once, or individually. The focus shifted from one person to another, then to the group, then to an individual. I had fantasized for a long time having sex with two women. The closer I came to doing it the more I realized that the real test would be how we dealt with each other afterwards. It worked out well. I had a lot of trust for my girlfriend before, and even more afterwards.

The best thing has been the pleasure my penis has given me. The worst was adultery. I wasn't happy in my marriage and got involved with another man's wife. It turned out to be terrible, and wasn't worth the few minutes of pleasure that resulted. It caused my lady, children, and the other couple a lot of pain. I would never do that again. Love does not commit adultery, destroy honor and cause pain.

The best thing is when I wielded my penis masterfully to please more than one woman at a time. It's when the pleasure is genuine and my needs come last. Being a good lover is all about pleasing my partner. I don't have pleasure if she's not pleased.

When I was in my early twenties and worked at a mental hospital, I attended a pretty woman who was suffering from the early stages of schizophrenia. I was asked to escort her to a changing room. She started taking off her clothes and just stood there. She looked so wonderful and ripe. The moment felt erotic, charged and forbidden. Wordlessly, we went at it right then and there. Afterwards I realized that she had not really consented and was in a powerless situation. In my mind it was like a rape. I've felt bad about it ever since. I don't know what happened to her later or where she is now. That was almost thirty years ago.

The best thing my penis did was to help create some beautiful human beings. It was such a pleasure making love without birth control and with the intention of creating life. It felt very freeing and cosmic, like what was happening was greater than our little bodies intertwined on the bed. Those kids are now young adults and may soon create children of their own. Raising them is the real hard part. That's where real devotion and love come in. Anybody can fuck and get pregnant. It's parenting that changes your life forever.

The worst thing I did with my penis was coerce my girlfriend to have anal sex when she didn't really want to try it. I kept bugging her over and over until she finally agreed.

I thought it felt great and said so. She said it was OK, but I could tell she was just trying to please me. I can usually tell when she has truly enjoyed herself and I could see she hadn't. She got up quickly and didn't want to talk about it. I should have listened to her, and not manipulated and cajoled to get my way.

My penis has given me something to hold onto. Something secure, reliable and trustworthy. I always know it's there waiting for me to grab it, give it a squeeze, or just say hello. It would feel funny to reach down and find nothing but space between my legs.

My penis was a bad, bad boy. When I was eleven years old I got mad at my father and peed in his shoes one night while he was asleep. When he put them on in the morning I heard him swearing through the walls. I remember him blaming the dog and hitting it on the nose with a newspaper. He never knew it was me.

The best thing my cock has done is give pleasure to other men's cocks and discover different ways to get off. Men know what other men want and like, and are willing to express it. Most of the time we don't even have to talk. We can tell by the other person's actions.

My dick just wouldn't wait. I was with the hottest chick I'd ever known and she was sucking and licking me all over and telling me how much she wanted me to fuck her. Before I knew what was happening I was coming all over her stomach. I was so close, yet so far. That didn't seem to stop her. She just kept going at it, fingering herself and getting me hard again. The next time, I got inside of her and was pumping away, but as soon as she started saying "Fuck me harder. Make me come," I came. She hadn't even gotten close to a climax and there I was shooting off inside of her and collapsing. I kept kissing her and licking her pussy until she came, but felt bad that we didn't come together when I was inside of her.

My wife calls my penis Willie. She says that Willie is the best thing that ever happened to her, besides me. Knowing she feels that way makes me feel real good about myself and my penis, and that's the best thing it's ever done.

The worst thing my penis has done is wander into other people's territory without taking precautions. I'd get so horny or drunk I wouldn't think about the consequences or how it would affect others, or me, in the future. I thought I had some magic immunity to catching or spreading diseases. That was in my teens, just five years ago, before I found out I had AIDS.

The best thing my cock has ever done is stay healthy. That old saying, "As long as you have your health," is true. And since my cock is so interwoven with the rest of my body, I've made it a point to keep my whole body and being as healthy as possible.

I was on some antidepressants for a while. They really helped with the depression, but had the side effect of making me impotent. I liked feeling better emotionally, but not being able to get an erection really affected my self-esteem. And I didn't want to take a second drug to counteract the side effects of the first. After six months I was able to slowly decrease the medication, feel emotionally balanced and enjoy sex again.

The most endearing quality of my penis is its ability to know when to pee and when to ejaculate. Thank God for the nerve endings that connect to that little valve at the base of my penis and tell it when to do which. I hate to think about what would happen without them.

PENIS FACTS

Will You Still Need Me When I'm Sixty-four?

A team of researchers from the University of Southern California has determined that "men and women are remarkably similar in their mating preferences." They found that college-age men and women prefer a long-term exclusive sexual relationship. Both sexes want a conscientious and compatible partner.

A cross-cultural questionnaire found that, contrary to popular misconceptions, over 80 percent of older women, and over 70 percent of older men, feel that sexual activity is important for health and well-being. Another survey found that 80 percent of married men over the age of 70, and 75 percent that were unmarried, remained sexually active.

It turns out that grandparents and college students want the same thing—love, commitment and sex. People of all ages enjoy one another's bodies and the pleasures, attachments and feelings that come with them.

If Your Penis Could Talk

Bouncing for Joy

I vividly remember the first time our body had a wet dream and I ejaculated on the sheets. He was dreaming that he was on a very large, naked woman's body bouncing up and down. Every time he landed he could feel her breasts around his head and me between her legs. We would bounce higher and higher, then plunge deeper and deeper. I don't think I've ever been as excited since, and that was forty years ago. For some reason nothing in our waking or sleeping state has ever matched the thrill of bouncing with pleasure, and falling towards that mass of warm, sensual flesh.

9

A Man's World

What are your experiences and observations about how men relate to one another in lavatories, locker rooms or public showers?

Author's note: *From what I've heard from my female friends, it seems that men and women are like night and day when it comes to their behavior in public, gender-segregated facilities.*

My over-riding observation is that men don't make eye contact in the bathroom—it's just not done. I don't know exactly why. I'm sure some of it's homophobia. We're taught that the individual is sacred and special, and you have to preserve that. Especially when it comes to your bodily functions—they shouldn't be shared with anyone. It follows that you avoid the other guy and don't talk.

There's wariness, like when two dogs come up, circle and smell each other. In a metaphorical sense, men are checking to see who has the bigger penis or the most power. We're checking one another to see who is a threat and who isn't.

When I was young—before puberty—and had just entered high school, we had to go in the locker room and strip for the first time in front of others. The seniors had hair, but some of the rest of us didn't. I would hold a towel in front of me. Later in life, I started going to nude beaches a lot, and that freed me up. Now when I go into the men's room, if a guy stands next to me to pee and starts looking at my penis, I leave real fast. I don't want to get near that energy.

I lament our culture of hyper-masculinity. I don't know why I'm saying that, other than the bathroom scenario represents a physical infrastructure or reminder of the utter compartmentalization of sexual function and emotion. You have steel and tile in there and they're both cold. And then there are the partitions. You have an exposed penis and the men are not looking at each other, or touching each other, or having fun with the absurdity of the situation. Everyone just pisses, washes his hands and asks about sports. It all reminds me of dismemberment.

The bathroom, with men holding themselves and pissing, reminds me of a personals ad I placed. In the ad I described myself as "unfortunately straight" because I don't get to experiment with the full range of sexual diversity. I'm stuck with my fucking heterosexuality. I appreciate the full range of expression and sexual orientation, but I can't go there because I'm a man.

It depends on why the men are in the locker room. I see them as jovial, not sexual.

It's a no-holds-barred in locker rooms. Women are talked about like pieces of meat—good tits, good ass, good fuck. But when you're with mixed company men don't talk like that. You clean up your act. I've seen men from other countries talk that way. They watch women come into work and rate them. It's a diversion. It's nice to fantasize. I think guys just like to look at women.

When I worked as a carpenter at a hospital, I got to know a lot of female nurses. They were very discreet, but when we came out of the bathroom they would stop us and tell more lewd jokes than anything I'd heard or seen in a men's locker room. I remember one cartoon a nurse had drawn. It showed a man standing naked with a noose around his neck and the rope going over a tree. The other end was tied to his cock. A woman was walking naked in front of him. The man was sweating because, as he watched her, his cock started to rise and he was about to hang himself. The nurse who drew it said, "See, see. You fuck with us and you fuck yourself."

I'm a member of a health club. I don't often change clothes there, but when I do I usually hear guys talking about very boring stuff. One guy will be sitting naked, while another is taking off his clothes, and they'll start talking about their wives or work in a way that gives mutual reassurance that they aren't gay. Talking that way makes them more comfortable. It seems like men need to establish what and who they are. I don't like men's locker rooms. I like sports, but I'm not a jock. I don't want to pretend that I'm comfortable showing my body to other men. It was like that in high school as well.

Men tend to do their thing and usually don't talk to other men while doing it. In locker rooms in high school or the army, I didn't think about or look at other men. I was afraid that if I did and happened to get an erection it would mean I was queer.

I remember, when I was young, frequently being amazed when in fancy hotels that there was a guy in the bathroom handing out towels, shining shoes and stuff like that. I always thought that was a strange job and was sure it was one I would never want to do.

In high school I always felt intimidated and thought I was a late bloomer. It seemed you were judged a lot on how you were developing physically. Guys would talk to each other and say things like,"You're a hairless wonder."

Once I went to a film festival and saw a film about a great Jewish baseball player. Afterwards, when I went to the bathroom, I heard a group of mostly Jewish men talking about their childhoods in Brooklyn. I loved listening to them, and realized what men missed by isolating themselves and not talking to each other. Recently, while attending a conference, I happened to run into the conference speaker in the bathroom. Instead of avoiding each other's gaze, we began talking and asking questions as we stood washing our hands side by side. It was immediate and intimate in a non-sexual and safe way.

I think a sense of exposure makes men hesitant to talk with one another in the restroom. Other men are a reflection of our own shit and stink. It hearkens back to our relationship with our fathers. Our fathers were the ones who, when we were little, helped take us into the bathroom and pull it down and out. And I don't think men usually have the time and attention to focus on such complex experiences.To talk with a strange man, let alone one you don't know, breaks the code of silence that most men follow.

The first time I went to a public school, in the seventh grade, we were obliged to take public showers after working out. I remember how easy some boys felt being naked in front of others. At the time, I attributed it to their being better hung or more endowed. I was acutely embarrassed by it all.

At school the neighbor boys would come into the bathroom and talk about their big pricks, girls and breasts, and tell nasty jokes all the time. I didn't join in because I hadn't had similar experiences. I started to feel uncomfortable and I didn't really enjoy talking like that.

When men are urinating at a common trough in a public bathroom, I notice there is almost no conversation. Part of that may be because peeing requires concentration. The whole experience of going to the bathroom has a private character to it. It's almost like it's in our genes to be like this. I knew one man who deliberately left the bathroom door open while he was going to the toilet. He felt it was important to overcome this taboo.

You're always checking out the size of your buddies, because prowess is associated with size.

I remember looking out of the corner of my eye every once in a while to see what other guys looked like. And now that I'm an adult I look to see if there's a cute guy that I'm attracted to.

I was always real self-conscious. I was a little overweight and compared myself to other guys to see who had a big dick. Everyone would take little side-glances, but never look directly at one another. Seeing someone who was not circumcised was rare in those days. I find that men rarely talk in the bathroom, let alone look at one another.

PENIS FACTS

What Are Your True Leanings?

In Kinsey's famous research on sexuality, he discovered that, viewed from above, 87 percent of erections were straight and the remainder curved to the side. Of the curved erections, four times as many curved left as curved right. There was no indication of what bearing this had on a man's politics.

If Your Penis Could Talk

The Ugly Duckling

When my life began I was very tiny and ugly. It took awhile to realize that I was exactly as I was supposed to be. For much of my life I didn't know that, despite my size, I was capable of doing all the right things, so I thought I was different. I thought there was no other penis like me in the world. I had a gigantic inferiority complex about my smallness. It wasn't something I felt I could talk about without the fear of being ridiculed.

I realized, much later in life, how perfect I really was. If I had known when I was younger, my early life would have been less miserable.

I also remember a most unpleasant event when I was older. I got an infection from the lady I was having sex with. It made me swell up and ache. At first I didn't know what in the hell was happening and thought if I got any bigger I'd detach and float away. We went to the health clinic, where they gave us some antibiotics. By the next day I was almost back to my normal size.

The final reassurance that my man and I were normal was when the woman we were having relations with became pregnant, which confirmed that everything worked just like it was supposed to. It was so reassuring that we made sure she got pregnant twice.

Now I've reached a level of satisfaction and understand that nothing major is going to change for the rest of my life. In spite of the bad start and the infection, most of my journey has been pleasant.

10

To Be or Not To Be

What are your experiences, thoughts, feelings and beliefs about circumcision?

Author's note: *Strong opinions prevailed, with little room for middle ground, doubt or questioning. Men were either against it or for it. Most of the American men I interviewed had been circumcised, and didn't feel as though they'd had much choice. They didn't know what it would be like to live with foreskin.*

It would have made my life easier if I had been circumcised, but on the other hand I feel I have a great deal of sensitivity in the head of my penis because I wasn't. I don't know why I wasn't circumcised, since most men of my generation were. Guys in the shower would make comments and jokes about me. I remember once pulling back the foreskin so I'd look circumcised.

The reason my father gave for my being circumcised was that he was circumcised, and that it was better health-wise.

I always thought it was a sexually repressive measure. You remove the skin and it creates scar tissue.

I'm not circumcised. I've heard a lot of the pros and cons. I don't think men should be circumcised as a standard practice. It doesn't seem fair to determine the amount of sexual feeling a man is going to have throughout the remainder of his life when he is a baby. My mother stopped the doctor from doing it to me, for which I'm grateful. I think some things that happen when we're babies stay with us, even if we aren't aware of them.

I'm against it. I spent a number of months naked on the sands of the Sinai and the tip of my penis got burned. If I'd had the foreskin I was born with that wouldn't have happend.

I'm of two heads about circumcision. I think an uncircumcised penis is rather ugly, but I'm concerned about the increasing evidence that circumcision is harmful. If forced to choose, I'd pick circumcision because it is better to look good then to feel good.

I don't know what it's like not to be circumcised. I think that young men can be cruel when it comes to pointing out differences. When I was young I wasn't picked on, but I might have been if I hadn't been circumcised.

I feel a little deprived that I never had a choice. My father said that circumcised were less likely to catch or pass on infections, but I will never know my natural state because I was circumcised without being asked about it. I've always heard that women prefer circumcised pricks, but I don't know why.

I'm very opposed to it. Here we are trying to raise a more sensitive generation of men and the first things we do is chop off the most sensitive part of their bodies.

I have no negative feelings about circumcision, but I did experience trauma when I was born and one of my testicles, which had not descended, was removed. It made me less sexual in a way, though theoretically it shouldn't. It made my scrotum smaller, which I think over the years has had a psychological impact.

I guess I'm for circumcision. It would be difficult to put it back on. It's probably all dried up and blown away by now.

I'm circumcised and I wish that I weren't. It's no big deal, but if I'd been given a choice I would not have been. I usually mention to friends who have sons that they might want to consider not circumcising them. Men tend to be less clean with their own bodies than women, and less intimate. The only thing I would be concerned about is uncircumcised men not cleaning themselves and how that would affect women. There are bigger issues and more painful things in life, but I don't think mutilation is helpful in any way.

I think it's unconscionable and barbaric. The act of circumcision is done without any thought, like some kind of ancient tradition. I wonder what the effects are. It doesn't seem healthy.

My generation was told, and I still believe, that circumcision is a must for keeping the penis clean. I feel sorry for men that have not had it done. I have zero religious feelings about it.

I was circumcised when I was six years old. My mother said she waited all that time because the doctor had changed his mind. I think it was because she noticed I had started playing with myself, and she didn't like it. As an adult I always wondered why. Both of my younger brothers were circumcised at birth. I think I have forgiven my parents for this action, but it clearly affected how I felt about myself. Three days after my circumcision the stitches broke and urination was very painful, so I had to be re-sutured. Since I wasn't given any real information about this event, I always thought there was something wrong with me and that I wasn't "right," especially in the area of sexual self-image. I felt damaged by that intervention. Though of all my siblings I am the best adjusted as an adult.

I don't see the purpose of it quite honestly. I think that to be the victim of circumcision must be a very painful experience for a young child. It's a ritual that doesn't serve much purpose.

Why would you cut anything off? I think it's ridiculous. You don't cut off someone's ears. Babies don't get to choose, either. Foreskin is also useful for masturbation.

I witnessed my son's circumcision. Seeing him strapped down in front of me and someone taking a knife to his penis was abhorrent. It seems like a superstition that isn't based on fact, and it's painful.

PENIS FACTS

Give Me Some Skin

Circumcision as a religious ritual is usually accompanied by celebrations: for Jews on the eighth day after birth and for Muslims within the first few years. Non-religious circumcision varies from one country to another and has changed with time. In England, it was fashionable in Victorian times. It is or was practiced among African Tribes, Australian Aborigines, and American Indians among others. Most baby boys in North America are circumcised. Most elsewhere are not. Worldwide about 20 percent of males are circumcised and 80 percent aren't.

Whether a male infant should be circumcised is an individual choice with no one right answer. Although it is no longer medically recommended that all newborn boys be circumcised, there are still some potential health benefits. Circumcision can help prevent infection and inflammation of the foreskin, as well as urinary tract infections. However, these problems can be avoided by good personal hygiene. Since it is easier to keep a penis clean and healthy with the foreskin removed, doctors do perform circumcisions on older children and adults with recurring infections. Circumcised men may be less likely to contract STDs, but safe sex and condoms are just as helpful.

Health practitioners who oppose circumcision believe the foreskin of the penis protects the penile glands from abrasion and friction; keeps the glands soft, moist and lubricated with oils; allows the natural development of the mucosal surface; protects infants' glands from infection; and aids masturbation, foreplay and intercourse.

Religiously oriented male circumcision will likely remain unchanged in the future, but the secular custom may decline. Nevertheless, arguments about the merits and demerits of the practice will doubtless continue unabated since removing the foreskin of the penis arouses strong emotions.

If Your Penis Could Talk

Getting Ripped

One upon a time, when I was eighteen, I had a most unpleasant experience. I got ripped in more ways than one.

We were having sex with our girlfriend and they were completely drunk, ripped, slashed, inebriated . . . whatever you want to call it. I was still working just fine though, standing up straight and ready to take what came.

She was getting down and seemed to want to eat me up like a cob of corn. She was sucking and licking and lightly biting me with her teeth. Then it happened. I could feel something tear. I don't think he felt it because he was so drunk, but they both heard it. They looked down and saw that the foreskin that attaches to my head had torn and was bleeding.

Like a fool, he wanted to keep going, but she was a little more cautious. After all, she didn't want to be taking in blood. They went ahead anyway and it didn't seem to phase any of us in the least. I healed quickly, within a day or two, and it's never happened since.

I'd be happier though if they didn't drink and fuck at the same time. I could have been split in two and they probably wouldn't have noticed.

11

Pissed Off

Has there ever been a time when someone touched your penis and you didn't want them too? If so, what happened and how has it affected your life?

Author's note: *It is now widely known that many women have been sexually, emotionally or physically abused or raped at some time in their lives. This reality is no longer denied, dismissed as a "private affair," or thought of lightly, due in large part to women like Ellen Bass and Laura Davis who showed the lifetime impact of such abuse in their book, The Courage to Heal. But even with such knowledge and public awareness, sexual abuse continues to injure and wound thousands of women.*

Even though I read the book, Victims No Longer, by Mike Lew, which details the stories of countless men who have been abused or raped and how they healed or lived with that reality, I still had not fully grasped the extent and impact of such violent acts on men's lives until I began asking this question.

When I moved to the states at age ten I was very introverted. One of the things that got me to come back again was bowling. I was in a program at an alley where there were forty lanes. There were about 2,000 kids in the program, which was run by a man named Bud, a single guy in his thirties.

Bud would often have kids over to his house after games to play cards and stuff. It turned out that he was a pedophile. I was at his house once, when I was about fourteen, playing cards. As the day went on I grew tired and took a nap on his couch. I remember waking up with him holding my erection in his hand and wiping me off. It was really strange. I had a lot of conflicted feelings, like confusion and frustration. It was exciting, yet didn't feel right. I didn't know how to talk about it to myself, let alone someone else. The worst repercussion was that I didn't want to be around Bud any longer and was perceived as being an ingrate—the kid who was rejecting Uncle Bud.

The other kids saw me not wanting anything to do with him. Up to that time I had wanted to become a professional bowler, but now that idea was all gone. I was castigated for walking out. A close friend of mine, who loved Bud, was about seventeen when I was fourteen. He didn't hear about Bud's abuse until Bud died and I told him about it. If Bud ever did anything to my friend, he never mentioned it. It happened so long ago. I don't think my sexuality is affected by those events in any way, but maybe there's something buried that I'm ignoring.

I had a homosexual experience when I was in my early teens. My family and a cousin's family went to North Carolina one summer. My cousin, who was two or three years older than I, was extremely sexual. Several times he suggested to me that we suck or beat each other off. He was constantly looking for an experience. In a tent one night, I went along with him. I masturbated him for a while and he masturbated me. I didn't want to orgasm because it would be too much, but I couldn't stop. It felt odd. It wasn't a welcome contact. Nowadays I'm not particularly comfortable when there are homosexual feelings and I'm the object of another man's desire, but I'm not sure how much that relates to that experience with my cousin.

I was traveling in Eastern Europe and went into a public restroom to use the urinal. A guy came up next to me, started jerking off, and said something to me in his language. I was grossed out by it and just left. That experience left a lasting imprint. Similar types of experiences or unwanted entrees create a kind of revulsion in me.

I was raped once. A very well dressed man in a suit started talking to me in Grand Central Station. I had been hitchhiking. He invited me out to see a movie, and after the movie he took me to his apartment. He asked if I'd ever taken Quaaludes, which I hadn't. He gave me some and then took me out drinking. I remember waking up in the middle of the night with a sharp pain in my ass. I was in in bed with this guy in a motel room. It was clear that he had raped me while I was unconscious. I had survived so much, hitchhiking that summer—it felt horrible to be taken advantage of just before I returned home. I didn't feel a sense of violation, because I was unconscious. I mostly felt stupid for getting myself into the situation. He was a bad person, but I blame myself for letting it happen. If I met him now I'd want to get him into a program, not punch him out.

I remember being in a hostel in Italy and the guy next to me asking if I wanted to sleep with him. I said no and he asked, "Why not?" He didn't bother me after that.

My father sexually abused me for many years as a child. It was especially hard to extricate myself, since it was happening right at home. There was nobody to tell in those days and nowhere to go. It was an untenable situation. I couldn't talk to my friends about it at school. My father was a well-respected member of the community and I didn't think anyone would believe me even if I said something.

The three most significant relationships in my life

have ended in part because of negative skills I learned in adolescence from my father's abuse. I learned how to survive an unwanted relationship, but not how to communicate or relate effectively. Since then I've been in a therapy a lot, and realize that I wasn't as mature as I thought I was. Each relationship has been a growth opportunity—a chance to change my habits and ways of being. I've learned how to talk about my childhood experience and that has helped. Still, I'm left with some mistrust towards women, wondering why my mother couldn't, or didn't, protect me from my father.

When I had a physical exam in high school the doctor checked my groin. I wasn't expecting that at all. I had no idea what was going on. After that I was always very leery of going to doctors.

There was a time I picked up a girl who was hitchhiking. She was a prostitute, but I didn't know it. She kept coming up with ways that I could spend money on her. She asked if I liked massage. Reaching into my crotch, she said, "I could give you a good massage, and I could even massage you down here." I remember feeling violated at the time. It gave me a brief glimpse at what women have to deal with repeatedly, being pawed and groped.

I have been with some women who wanted to be sexual when I didn't, but those times were rare.

I didn't want to be bathed. I was very young and that part of my body was "mine." I didn't want my mother to touch me there.

When I was fifteen a man who was in his twenties said he loved me.There were times when he gave me pleasure, but sometimes I said no, and he honored that and stopped. I wasn't molested, but boundaries were crossed. He didn't discuss what he was going to do before he did it. It wasn't natural for me, because I'm heterosexual, but at the time I was confused. One of the good things about that relationship was that it made me think critically about how relationships are initiated, how sex is begun, and whether and how to talk about it. Since then I have talked with my women lovers about these issues.

I don't recall ever being touched when I didn't want to be, but that doesn't mean it never happened.

I remember a man (a trusted philosophy professor) making advances and telling me he would love to fondle me. It came at a time when I was grieving the breakup of a relationship with my girlfriend. I no longer trusted him after that, and let him know that I didn't want him to touch me in any way.

It happened to me in the Boy Scouts. A scoutmaster slipped into our tent, supposedly to check and make sure we were OK. He really creeped me out. What he did was shocking and confusing. He molested me in other environments as well, but I don't want to talk about it. At that age I felt very victimized.

Because of things that happened to me as a child, I am more aware of attractions between men. While they are not readily accepted, I realize that they do exist, and I feel more prepared to respond in ways that are not hurtful to the other person, but make it clear that I don't consent.

When I was in a human sexuality class, the women in the class did an experiment. They had me and the only other man in the class walk between them while they looked only at our crotch and butt. It felt very uncomfortable and helped us understand a little bit of what women experience all the time.

When I was about 12 years old and on a church ski trip, a man who talked real nice during the day came into my dorm at night, woke me up and said he wanted me to go with him. I said no, and he proceeded to put his hand down inside my sleeping bag. I kicked him and yelled and he left. I told my parents about it when I got home. They didn't do anything about it, except say I did the right thing. Who knows how many other boys he fondled or abused? Ever since then I've been a little leery of men.

PENIS FACTS

Help Stop the Cycle

Our mothers, sisters, lovers, aunts, grandmothers and daughters shouldn't have to live with the fear of rape, but they do. Women are usually raped by someone they know—a partner, husband, father or uncle. Home can be the most violent place in America. Men are less likely to be raped, but when they are it is usually by a stranger—someone outside their family or work environment.

Sexual assault is not an act of sex. It is a brutal act of violence. It is sex without permission. It is an act of dominance and power.

"Rape jokes" are an oxymoron. There's nothing funny about rape.

You can prevent abuse and rape by examining your own attitudes, paying attention to the language you use to refer to women (sexual objects can turn into sexual targets) and talking with other men about it. Report abuse and help prevent others from being abused. Stop harassment and speak up when you witness it. Don't tolerate sexual abuse in any way, shape or form—period.

If Your Penis Could Talk

The Proof Is in the Pudding.

When my man, Elijah, was a young kid he heard horrible stories about boarding schools and headmasters. Other kids told him that the headmaster put salt peter (potassium nitrate) in their pudding in order to keep them from being sexually active.

Elijah, being a scientific kind of guy and not wanting to wait to find out if the stories were true, tried a little experiment before being sent off to join his brother at a live-in institution. He was lucky enough to have access to all the materials he needed, since his father was a chemist and had been teaching him chemistry since before he could walk.

Elijah got hold of some salt peter and took large amounts for a number of days. After two weeks he discovered that I was still able to get hard in spite of the potassium nitrate. Thus his fears of boarding school were alleviated. Even though he stopped taking the chemicals after that, he continued to stroke me daily, just to make sure everything was all right.

12

Another Lifetime to Learn

If reincarnation were a reality, would you choose to come back as a man or a woman, and why?

Author's note: *Though a slight majority of men definitely wanted to be reborn male, quite a number said they would like to see what life would be like as a woman, and most had some curiosity about the physical and emotional experiences of the opposite sex.*

Definitely male. Women are fucked up and crazy. In my experience the concept of women being more in touch with their feelings can easily go overboard and be just as troublesome in relating as men being out of touch. We need some sort of emotional hermaphrodite middle ground.

I'd like to be a woman. I've done it as a man and it would help in relating to others to know what it's like as a woman. To experience childbirth must be quite awesome.

I'd want to come back as a man because I don't think I've learned all I need to know about being a man. I'd like another lifetime to get it better. I have a lot of regrets, and I'd like to try a different way of being.

I would want to be a woman. Basically, we're all human beings and we all have the same needs and desires. Males and females just interpret things differently. I think women are more in touch with their feelings and able to express them. Men seem more involved in the material world. I'd like to see what it's like having an orgasm as a woman, over and over.

My perception is that men in general have better advantages in life—the best seat, metaphorically speaking. In many ways it seems it would be more difficult as a woman, for example, to always be the object of men's lust. In many societies, including ours, women are still second class citizens.

In the context of dicks, I suppose I would come back as a desirable man. The probable range of sexual experiences is greater. It's a strange thing to think about. I was going to say a desirable woman, but that would mean I wouldn't get to experience the roving, chasing part of being male. I think women are more the chased than the chasers, and there is something unique about being on the prowl.

The older I get the more I realize that women don't look at men in terms of physical beauty. If I reincarnated as Antonio Banderas, or some rock star who gets pussy any time he wants it, my desirability would still depend on exuding something else. There's some rider attached to male desirability. I am willing to acknowledge the socially constructed nature of virtually everything, except when it comes to male and female differences. I don't fully buy into the argument that it's all culturally learned.

I don't know if women want the same thing as men, or something else, but I do know that they want more. As a man, I'm willing to take a nice sweet hard body, bend it over, fuck it and be happy for life. A woman wants the sex along with looks and a personality, and will take a charming personality over a pretty face or big cock.

Definitely as a woman. I would want to see how the other half lives. I've always suspected that the differences between sexes are not that great. For the first thirty years of my life I had a sense of myself as a person, not as a man. Again and again I would find myself talking with women about emotions and relationships. Other men didn't do that. Women are willing to get together in groups and talk about feelings. I enjoy that. When I was thirty I did a program with some other guys. One guy, who was fifteen years older than me, said, "You have no idea what it is like to be a real man." It hurt, but I felt his assessment was accurate. In the last ten years I've had more of a sense of what being a man is all about. To me it means being a provider and caring for women and children.

I would come back as a woman. Partly because of the novelty and partly because I've always had a fantasy of being the other half of the sexual combination. Each gender has its unique difficulties and crosses to bear. As a woman, it seems like you could always find someone to have sex with you. As a man that's not so true. In most societies women are less appreciated, though I think women as a group have a stronger sense of kinship among themselves. I wish men could relate more like women do, on a less superficial level. They want to know how you are, how you're feeling. I wish men were more like that.

It would be difficult to switch. There are times when I just want my woman, when I feel like being aggressive, more centered in my lust. In the past I lacked the self-confidence to feel I was attractive enough for a woman to lust after me. Once I felt better about myself, those doubts arose less often. I began to see that some women I met were more desperate for me than I was for them. That made me feel that I was a powerful individual, and that I knew how to please and take care of a woman. It made me feel good about being a man.

That would be a tough choice. I think I might choose to come back as a woman in order to have a different experience. I see a lot of pros and cons on both sides. Men have a lot more strength and opportunities than women, but with these come the responsibility to be a bread-winner. Being able to experience giving birth and being a mother would be cool, but, god it's got to hurt. Being taken care of would be nice, but without having to give up my independence and freedom. Being a mother, so heavily depended upon in such a primal way, would be difficult. It's like there is no rest.

My first thought is that I'd want to come back as a man. I've enjoyed being a man. I think a lot of it has to do with the cultural bias around women and the cultural power that men still have in our society. I think that's the major reason. The thought of having a menstrual period once a month isn't very appealing. And the thought of a penis coming at me doesn't jive. I'm sure that women who have achieved some balance in their lives are probably satisfied with being a woman.

I think I would come back as a woman. I'd do it for the change, to be able to give birth and have another life growing inside of me. Also being able to fully embrace my nurturing and emotional side, without any conflicting emotions. When men do that, they face criticism and judgment, both externally and internally. Men aren't expected to be as emotionally aware and open as women.

A man. I've always done anything I wanted to do. There are no roadblocks. Nothing has gotten in the way. Women get stereotyped a lot, and I don't believe they have the same opportunities.

I would rather be born a female in the next life because I want to know the world differently. Objectively, men and women are not that different, but how we relate to, work with, and exploit the world is very different. In certain species of animals, males show some of the worst behavior towards females.

To experience the world as a woman would be very frightening. I'd want to have other women around me, to be close with women in a way that was not narrowly, sexually defined. I'm not gay, but I know gay men who seem to have more access to the intellects of women than heterosexual men do, and they don't seem to have to work for years to figure women out. As I get older I find that talking with women and reading authors like Bell Hooks has helped me to knock down my own oppressive thinking. I believe that the world could be more equal if women had more power and gender differences were less important. How we define human relations and how we raise children and families is more important than gender.

I would take the luck of the draw. It might be interesting to feel what it's like to give birth and to bleed. I have attended three births and they were awesome. My wife says it feels like a great relief when her period starts. Of course, I am painting a romantic picture. I know that birth is also painful, and there is nothing like a flood in the underwear or menstrual cramps to make a period feel like a bummer.

It also might be interesting to be the sex object, rather than the aggressor. As a man, I always think about making love, but whether I get to or not is often dependent on the willingness of my wife. When you're not married, you are looking for a woman willing to make love with you. It might be interesting to be a woman and call the shots. Most women can make love almost any time they want.

I've always wondered how much of myself I've constructed. Part of developing a relationship with myself is becoming compassionate towards those parts of myself that are more classically male, that I see mirrored in other men. I don't turn away from other men who behave like louts.

In my bravest times, I'd like to come back as a male, however not right away. First there needs to be more advancement in the species. To come back as a male would help me to get to know myself better, and not spend the first part of my life dealing with whatever mandate I've been handed. I'd like to not buy into the twin requirements and expectations of success and survival, and not do so much damage to myself and others.

Men are still trying to form community and I'd want to help hasten that. I would not presume that women have it easy. One thing that triggers me is when people try to engage in gender essentialism. I find that very off-putting. I was walking behind a local restaurant recently and heard a couple of women telling each other, "All men are like that." I said, "Well, that's quite a generalization."

If I came back as a woman, it would feel like an abandonment of the species, of men's work in progress. It's like always wanting to be some place that you aren't.

I think I would come back as a man because women take more abuse than men do. They have to work harder for everything. I don't think I'd want to be pregnant and put up with that. I have fantasized what it would be like to have sex as a woman and feel some attraction to the passivity. That would be the only desirable reason to come back as a woman, because passivity in a woman is sanctioned. Of course that is my stereotype of a women's sexual experience.

I'd like to be both. I know this is a male perception, but I'd like to have the woman's nurturing point of view, which to me seems more fluid and non-Euclidian and open. It's not like the straight line of putting the tractor in gear and plowing the field. I like lightness, and as a male I feel sort of like a heavyweight. I'd like to be a butterfly.

As a male, I like building things, figuring things out and designing things. I like challenges in nature and a certain amount of physical hardship. I like getting grungy and crusty. I love going off into the wilderness for six weeks and seeing what's over the next hill and having nobody tell me what to do or not do.

13

Another Lifetime to Learn
Women Choose

If reincarnation were a reality, would you choose to come back as a man or a woman, and why?

Author's note: *Unlike the men, the women that replied to this question had little doubt. They all want to come back as women. They didn't hesitate with their answers and said they'd be surprised if a woman wanted to be a man. Here's why.*

I think women are stronger and have more sympathy and empathy. The only reason I'd come back as a man is because it's easier to go pee somewhere when you're traveling.

A woman. Women are more grounded in their views and thoughts, and have a more wholesome attitude towards all people and both sexes. We don't have testosterone, which eliminates a lot of ego-tripping.

I'd come back as a woman because I don't know anything else. I love being feminine, which to me means the ability to be a mother, not just to children but to the earth. I'd miss that nurturing feeling. Nurturing feels like compassionate caring. I wouldn't want the strife men have. They always seem to be measured by their financial worth and I wouldn't want that pressure. It seems like the self-worth of every man I've ever met is caught up in what they've accumulated.

I'd want to be a woman. I like feeling feminine. I think a woman's body is sexier than a man's body. Women are more sensual and beautiful. We can do things to enhance our beauty that are culturally acceptable. Most men can't or won't do those things. Women can transform themselves. We have choice. I don't think there's that big a difference emotionally or mentally between women and men.

I'd want to come back as a woman, for personal growth. We have more ways to experience pleasure, peace and other feelings. We are able to give birth and to nurture. I think there are brain differences between men and women. I don't think our behavior is all culturally learned. I think men have it harder and they are much more vulnerable with regard to their sex parts.

A woman, because I don't want to be an oppressor. If I came back as a man, in our culture with its present role restrictions, my quality of life would be limited. I wouldn't be able to be intimate or feel as much. And I wouldn't trade that for male privilege or power.

Women rock. Men sit around and physically or emotionally pound their chest saying, "Look at me." They seem so self-centered and unaware of their surroundings. If that's what it's like as a man, there's no way I'd want to go through that. It must be very boring and monotonous. Women get to change constantly. We can go through a million seasons all in one day. Change and fluidity aren't so threatening to us since we have to deal with them physically all our lives.

Without a doubt, I'd come back again as a woman. I love making love to a woman as a woman. It's like seeing and touching myself. We know each other so well. We know what makes us tick and turns us on. Most men seem clueless when it comes to sex. They just want to get off. They're so linear. We like to ebb and flow, rise and fall and make circles out of life and love.

I've always wondered what it's like to have something hanging between your legs that feels so driven and out there, but I've never thought about it enough to want to come back as a man. It's only been a passing question. It must be kind of weird to be born with a penis. Of course, I guess it would feel weird to a man not to have a dick and balls hanging there. What can I say?

I enjoy complexity and interconnections. I experience women as complex, for the most part, and men as simple. I know that's a generalization and there are exceptions, but generally it holds true. It usually doesn't take me long to figure out a man. Women can take an entire lifetime.

If I could choose to be a man, with all the privileges and power they have had over women for centuries, I don't think I would. I couldn't live with myself knowing what my gender had done and was doing to so many people in the world. I know some women have been just as cruel and thoughtless, but if you look at history, and at how women live in many countries now, you see that it is usually men who have put them down, abused them, or controlled everything they do. If I could come back and be like some of the men I know personally, the ones who pay attention to their behavior, thoughts and feelings and take responsibility for themselves, then maybe I'd consider it, but even then I'm not sure.

I'd never want to give up the experience of giving birth, nursing and raising children. I know men can raise children too, and there are some wonderful fathers out there, but they can't get pregnant, carry a child, or know what it's like to have a human being come out of your body and depend on you to survive. It's overwhelming, mystical and indescribable, and it's something almost all women can relate too.

PENIS FACTS

Penis Thief

Just a few years ago police in Lagos, Nigeria, arrested a woman who had been accused by an angry crowd of stealing a man's penis with witchcraft. Without any evidence, the police took her away, sparing her further insults and beating from the crowd. It has long been believed in Nigeria that witches can steal men's sexual organs with just a handshake or an incantation.

Is this another blatant example of men's fear of the creative power of women? It seems that when men feel inadequate, out of control or weak, they often blame women instead of acknowledging their own feelings and taking responsibility for themselves. I believe the reverse of Freud's old adage and paternalistic theory about "penis envy." It is not women who envy men, but men who envy women. Men have "womb envy." Because we cannot experience the ultimate act of creation, giving birth, we try to control those that can, and are in fact jealous of such powers. You can see this dynamic acted out daily when men try to create, control and manipulate others. Most men do not admit to such feelings, but as Freud used to say, it's all in the unconscious mind, whether we are aware of it or not.

If Your Penis Could Talk

Painful Withdrawal

My master Mark and I once went on an unexpected, but necessary, adventure. He was put under anesthesia for a surgery that lasted seven hours and a catheter had to be inserted in me. He didn't feel a thing when it went in, but I was cringing. After the surgery, when they took it out, there were some unexpected difficulties. We didn't realize anything was amiss until we got home and masturbated. For three days after that we couldn't pee without experiencing an extraordinary amount of pain.

Look Dad, No Hands!

Phil used to work as a woodcutter out in the poison oak infested woods. It took him awhile to figure it out, but he eventually learned how to pee without handling me. Thank God. Before he got the knack of peeing with no hands he'd put me out of action for weeks.

So Nice Out This Morning.

My man is blond and prone to sunburn. Back in '66 we went to a state park and heard about a beach nearby that was clothing-optional. He got stoned and took me down to the beach, where he proceeded to take off all his clothes and put on suntan lotion. He put it everywhere except on me because he didn't want people to think he was playing with himself in public.

I hadn't seen sunlight in years. Within fifteen minutes I was turning pink. I tried to get his attention, but he was too stoned to notice. Another fifteen minutes went by and I was one roasted wiener.

It was the worst burn I'd ever gotten. He could hardly wear pants for a week after that sunny day, and when he did he kept them so loose they almost fell off.

14

Women's Reactions to Cocks

When you hear the word penis, what kind of thoughts, feelings and reactions do you have?

Author's note: *Men orchestrate their relationships and reactions to many life situations based on their perceptions of what we believe women want, expect or desire from us. Some of our behavior and deeds match those perceptions. At other times we don't have a clue what women are thinking about or how they feel about our bodies, especially our penis. If we really want to listen and know, here's an opportunity to find out.*

My sex-ed teacher standing in front of the class and my husband going, "Yep, yep, yep—there she blows."

Makes me think of how men are so proud of it.

I think of being horny, of sex, love, and masculinity, and of men thinking they're powerful and in control.

It makes me think of one word descriptions—male, fun, sex, softness, hardness, erect, playfulness, admiration, sensual and arousal.

I think of an excited erection. It feels charged and full of energy. I call it "our friend Dick."

Pesky, powerful and aggressive. Something that wants to do it all the time, even when you're tired.

It makes me giggle.

It can be dangerous and cause pregnancy or disease.

It's like a leash. You can lead them around with it.

A class of their own.

A headache.

Cock-a-doodle do.

Pleasure. I like it.

It's like a thermometer, checking the temperature of the waters.

Penis is a terrible name for it. There should be a better word.

An ugly, but useful tool. Yuck!

Bill Clinton and Antonio Banderas.

Men. Sex. Power. Secrecy. Taboo-ness. The sexual experience. It's connected with a power image of men. There's some kind of negotiation with power. My relationships have been pleasurable and exciting. Power is out there to be grabbed—to be negotiated. I had to learn what I wanted out of men and whether I was getting that or not. Letting them know that my desire, request or demand should be listened to and that it's important.

A good towel rack.

I wonder what it feels like to have one. What it is like when it's hard? I think of force and insistence. Even though I grew up with three brothers and my dad, I never saw a penis until I was eighteen. It was surrounded in mystery. I think my mom told me or gave me the impression that if you got them excited they were uncontrollable and had to have their way, sort of like an alcoholic who can't stop drinking.

A boyfriend told me that it was physically painful for men if they had an erection and then didn't have an orgasm. I believed him and thought it was my responsibility to take care of his penis by helping him come—so it wouldn't hurt.

I always wished that God would have made semen so it wouldn't get so cold so fast when it's outside the body. Rolling onto cold cum on the sheets is always a shock.

I think of the penis as semen's messenger.

The penis is a good thing. A good feeling. Intimacy, touch and connection.

It makes me think of war, testosterone, and being taken advantage of, as well as my first boyfriend.

It's interesting to look at, but the size doesn't make any difference when it's being used.

It's not something that is appealing to me, but connected to a human being it's always something that's been beautiful.

It signifies centuries of oppression for women and male patriarchy. It's like a weapon of war.

A sense of knowing there's vulnerability in having external genitalia, in being exposed. A dual feeling of strength and vulnerability.

My pulse leaps with alarm when you say, "penis." It signals iffy ground, and most often it signals prurient, disturbing conversation. It creates instant tension. I feel a red flag go up, that I need to pay attention.

My initial reaction is one of poor associations. My father was a philanderer and my ex-husband was a womanizer. I think men have no intelligence or thought of the damage that can be done, of children that can be made. I think we are a very immature society in terms of sexuality.

All men's egos and how they associate their penis with their ego and measure themselves as a human. I think a lot of it is inherited in their biological makeup. Our society feeds that stereotype, but it also seems like a physical reality.

PENIS FACTS

The Best Sex

Lovemaking implies giving, receiving and sharing pleasure, not performing, exercising or proving endurance.

Satisfaction Guaranteed

A number of studies show that men have better, more satisfying sex with their spouse then they do with their mistress.

If Your Penis Could Talk

The Power Switch

I used to think I had great powers and could control women with this little thing when I'd get hard and rise up. I always took control on dates. I was all my man thought about when he was younger and with girls.

As we both aged, our sense of control changed and we learned how to be patient and quit trying to manipulate and have sexual control or power. It was scary at first, but now it's become quite freeing.

Rising to the Occasion

When I was a teenager I had a lot of energy and liked sticking my nose around. I liked to play. Now that I'm in my early twenties, moving on in my life and maturing as a dong, I'm learning to see the finer things—to slow down a bit, take my time and keep exploring. I hope there will be a point where I meet another shlong that I can be content with for the rest of my life.

Longing

My guardian, Chang, has had his heart broken a number of times when he was in love with women, but they weren't in love with him. He even got married and expected to be with his wife for the rest of his life. It took us many years to recover from the divorce, and made us not want to commit to another relationship. He tried to protect himself from getting hurt again by having casual, meaningless affairs. We were an equal opportunity employer and never discriminated.

But these affairs always left him feeling empty. It was becoming an addiction, a way to numb out. How much sex could we have? How long could we stay up screwing without sleeping? The lustful aspects were exciting and the supposed "conquests" were a thrill, but after the sex was over there was nothing there.

PENIS FACTS

Lovemaking Olympics

Recent research legitimizes sex as a healthy form of exercise on a par with running, walking or swimming.

Some specialists in cardiovascular disease have found that having sex three to five times a week can cut the risk of a stroke or major heart attack in half!

A study of 2,400 men in the town of Caerphilly, Wales, discovered that those who had three or more orgasms a week had half the number of strokes or heart attacks as those who didn't. The study lasted for ten years.

It turns out that even mild or moderate forms of physical activity, including sex, can help protect the heart and decrease the chance of illness.

15

Penis to Penis

If you had a son, what would you want him to know about his penis?

Author's note: *Though most of the men I spoke with reported that their fathers had talked with them little, if at all, about sex, their body, or their penis, they all had clear ideas about what information should be passed on to a son. However, the majority of the fathers who were asked this question admitted that they had not spoken to their sons about sex, and in that sense seemed to be repeating the behavior of their fathers.*

My son is about seven and a half and plays with himself all the time. He's always been curious why he wasn't circumcised as I was. After a shower one day, he pointed at my penis and said, "Why did they do that?" He's more aware of himself at seven then I was at eighteen. He asked about sex and how we mate. I let him know that it's OK to ask. I don't want him to feel ashamed like I did growing up. I don't want that kind of energy to spill onto him.

I have a grown son. I don't recall our ever talking about it one way or another. An awkwardness about sexuality has always existed between us.

It would be nice if there were something institutionalized that provided kids the opportunity to have a discussion with a parent or parent figure about sex. It's not something I would go up and start talking about. With all the sex education we supposedly have in this modern age, I don't recall ever hearing or talking much about it in school.

I'd want my sons to know that sexual exploration of themselves is a good, normal, healthy thing, and that asking questions about themselves is good too. They shouldn't feel ashamed about it.

I would like my sons to know that their bodies are beautiful and be able to come talk with me about any questions they have regarding their sexuality. In practice it almost never happens, but I'd like them to be able to talk about the naturalness of our bodies.

I'd want my son to know the hazards involved—the diseases, how they are transmitted and the steps that can be taken to prevent them. My son didn't start talking about his penis much until he was in his twenties.

My son had his first girlfriend this summer and it provided a great opportunity to talk with him about sex and relationships. We have discussed sex, what he's thinking and experiencing, and any questions he has—and will continue to do so.

I was always hiding my urges as a young adult. There wasn't anything beautiful about it then and I don't want to pass on that guilt.

I think the things I talk about with my daughter are the same I'd be emphasizing with a boy. Your body is your own. It's under your control and you can do with it as you choose. Other people aren't allowed to touch you unless you want them to. And encouraging her to say no, and giving her the words to do so. Letting her know that there are boundaries.

I think kids get more information in school then we got.

I guess I'd want him to have fun with it, be open about it, and not feel strange or bad about exploring his penis and what it's for and what it can do. I'd want him to be comfortable with it.

I want him to honor all his partners. I believe my sons need to live their own lives. I'm not trying to live vicariously through them. I believe everything will be provided to them. I don't try to control or lecture them. It's not about telling them what to do with their penis, it's about setting an example by the way I use mine. And I try to treat others with honor.

He should become aware of what is driving the show, his penis or his head, and then decide which he wants to listen to. The best way I can think of to teach him is by example, by showing how I treat women. I hope, too, that when opportunities come up he will be open to talking about them.

I do have a son. I have been, and will continue to be, absolutely honest with him about what I've done in my life. It is such a central part of who I am that I can't imagine foregoing whatever good can come from sharing my experiences with my son. I consider my son to be a very well balanced and healthy individual. He knows that my partner's and my sexuality, and how we express it, has nothing to do with our love and commitment towards him. I feel confident in sharing that with him and know it won't hurt him, but will give him what I didn't have growing up—not because my parents were bad, but because of the social protocol they followed.

I'd want him to know that his penis is OK and to be uninhibited about his sexuality. I don't mind being naked. I have no embarrassment about it and I'd like him to have the same comfort with his body, masturbation and sex in general. I want him to be comfortable being an animal.

I'd want him to know as much as I could impart, to the best of my ability. I'd want him to know that it's a part of his body to be respected and not feared. It requires attention. Mostly, I'd want to be available to help him understand.

I'd want him to know that there are a lot of normal feelings that revolve around his penis and that shame shouldn't be one of them. I'd also try to get him to connect his penis to his brain, and act with as much thought as possible. I'd want him to respect women.

We never talked about sex because it felt uncomfortable. I want him to be careful, though, and to take precautions so he doesn't get AIDS.

I want him to know that his body is protected by his mother and me, and loved and known. He can learn to love and know his own body, in terms of accepting and enjoying and playing. I want him to know that his genitals are the genitals of a boy who will become a man, and that they have specific functions, one of which is sexual. In friendships and relationships, he should not only be careful of himself but of the other person.

The penis is tender and can be hurt, so you need to be careful with it, though it is not as important to protect as your eyes, head and hands. You can't hurt your penis unless you have an accident.

A son should learn that a penis is a body part that's no different than other parts and is nothing to be ashamed of. He should know what it does, in every capacity, and how it affects his thoughts.

That it is a magnificent creation and he can define his own relationship to it. It has a powerful presence in his life and the life of others. And with it goes responsibility.

That it is not dirty, the source of evil or embarrassment or shame. It's also not a weapon or a means of domination. There are far more important things in life than its size or function. A priest once asked a class, "If you have sex for ten to twenty minutes a day for the rest of your life, what will you do with the other twenty-three hours and forty minutes a day?" It put a lot more value on the rest of life and helped lessen the importance and dominance of sex in our culture. That is an idea I'd want to pass on.

I'd tell him not to be led by it. I assume that he would need to learn how I handled sexual issues, and then hope that he would find what was right and appropriate for him.

I'd want him to be conscious of it. I'd want him to feel free to get to know it better and to use it for the betterment of humanity and not just himself.

My son is 24 now. I'd tell him to be more mindful where he puts it. If he were open to it I'd discuss the difference between love and sex.

PENIS FACTS

Recommended Daily Allowance

Semen is a mixture of sperm and fluids from the seminal vesicles and prostate. The prostate fluids include prostaglandin, water, sugar and minerals such as calcium and zinc. The amount of semen ejaculated is approximately 1 teaspoonful, depending on the frequency of orgasm.

Where you deposit your daily teaspoon of orgasmic fluids depends on your habits, your partner, and the consequences you wish to avoid or create.

This mixture of fluids is not recommended as a replacement for a healthy diet and does not supply the recommended daily allowances of calcium, zinc and water the body needs, though it could be offered as an enjoyable supplement or salty treat.

If Your Penis Could Talk

Use Me in Sacred Ways and Pray I Don't Dribble

I believe life is sacred. May we all feel our blessedness and not our shame. I will use my energy to create spiritual bliss with the one I love or with myself. I will bring heaven from my roots to the top of my limb. I will stand up to show my appreciation for the gods of lust, pleasure, devotion and tantric loving.

I pray that my urination will flow freely and with ease. I hope I will not dribble too much as I age and, if I do, may I continue to remember to love myself and the body I'm attached to regardless of it's functioning state. We are all from mother earth.

PENIS FACTS

Nature's Call

During the times of the Roman Empire they used words from nature to describe the penis, such as *arbor* (tree), *thysus* (stalk), *falx* (sickle), and *radix* (root). Semen was *ros* (dew).

Keep that in mind the next time you go for an early morning walk in the woods. Imagine that towering penises surround you, with semen dripping from their leaves like dew. Then again, you might just see a bunch of old trees standing around with drops of water evaporating in the sun.

If Your Penis Could Talk

The Primeval Ooze

I have been to many wonderful places. The happiest place on earth is where it's warm.

I fully realized who I was on a hillside on a warm summer day when nobody was around and my friend showed me the sun and made me weep.

I have found that the place that is warmest doesn't have much light.

I have a place that is my home, a place where I am bathed in fragrant liquid of the one whom I knew first, when I was born.

This dark warm fragrant place and flowing liquid are forever new. They come from an ancient memory of my very beginning when I first saw the light.

It wasn't home, but a new place I wanted to visit again and again and again. I want to keep the memory as close as possible without being cleansed.

One way or another, other people need to know that all of us, male and female, have come from that same place.

PENIS FACT (OR FICTION?)

Boxing Masculinity

Masculine is defined as something that is "characteristic of men and boys, as strength, vigor, boldness, etc.; manly; virile."

- Should masculinity be defined so narrowly?
- Is one's masculinity judged solely by "strength, vigor and virility?" If so, has it always been judged that way?
- Do one's masculine traits stay fixed and static or are they changeable and adaptive?
- Is our masculinity predetermined by genetics?
- Is there one masculinity or are there many?
- Does one's masculinity change with age?
- How does one's social, economic, geographical or cultural environment influence one's perception of what it means to be masculine?
- Do gay men define or demonstrate masculinity differently than straight men?
- Do men express masculinity differently with different people, *e.g.,* wife, children, male friends?
- Does simply having a penis make one masculine?

Think twice before you attach yourself to someone else's definition of masculinity and allow it to dictate how you act, what you do or who you are.

16

A Warm Penis Farewell

This marks the end of our exploration of what men think and feel about their penis, what they experience with their penis, and how those things affect their perceptions of themselves, others and the world in which they live.

It has been a pleasure sharing these stories, facts, observations and insights into the male psyche, and discovering common ground while celebrating differences. Though this brings us to the end of our journey, I hope it is also a beginning.

Take these words to heart, share them with others, and continue *The Penis Dialogues* with the men and women who are part of your life. Continue to look honestly at your thoughts and behaviors, and make wise choices for yourself and those you love. And wherever your path leads you, remember to handle it with care.

About the Author

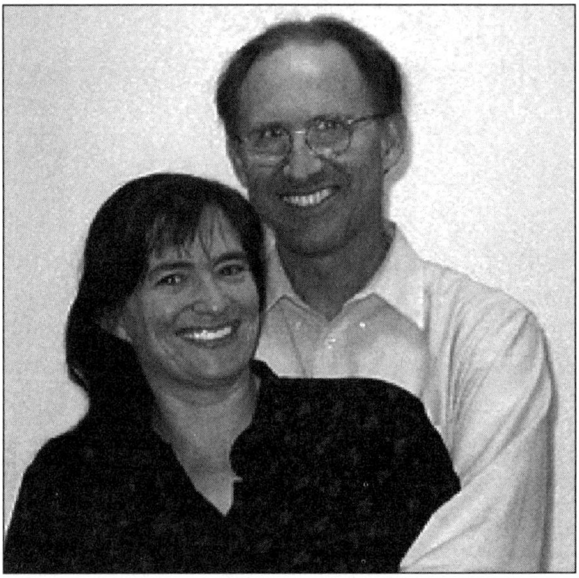

—Shona Constans Blumeneau

Gabriel Constans, Ph.D., shown here with his wife Audrey Blumeneau, is a Santa Cruz Sentinel columnist and a grief counselor with Hospice Caring Project. He has been a mental health and drug abuse counselor, social worker, nursing assistant and hospital chaplain. Author of seven books published in the U.S., his articles appear worldwide in magazines, journals and newspapers. He is the father of five children.

Gabriel Constans can be contacted at:
Web Site: www.gogabriel.com
Email: constans@gogabriel.com

Titles Published by Aslan

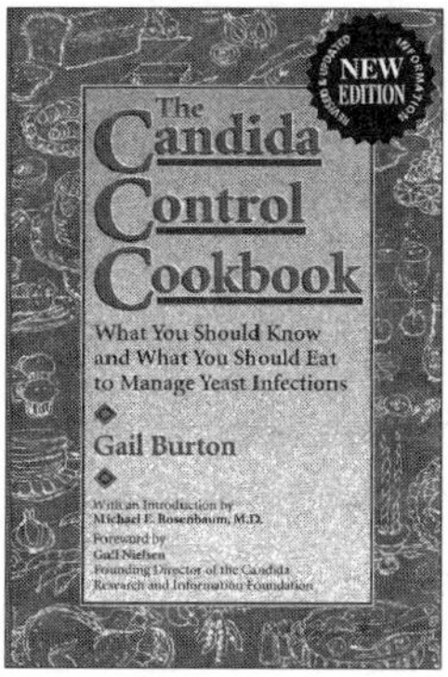

The Candida Control Cookbook What You Should Know And What You Should Eat To Manage Yeast Infections
by Gail Burton
$14.95
ISBN 0-944031-67-6

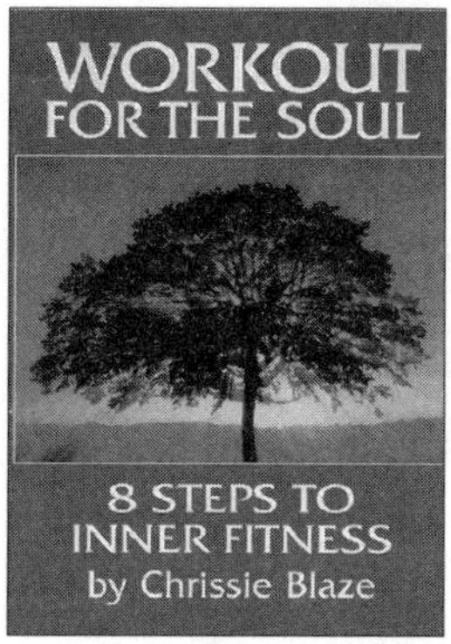

Workout for the Soul: 8 Steps to Inner Fitness
by Chrissie Blaze
$14.95
ISBN 0-944031-90-0

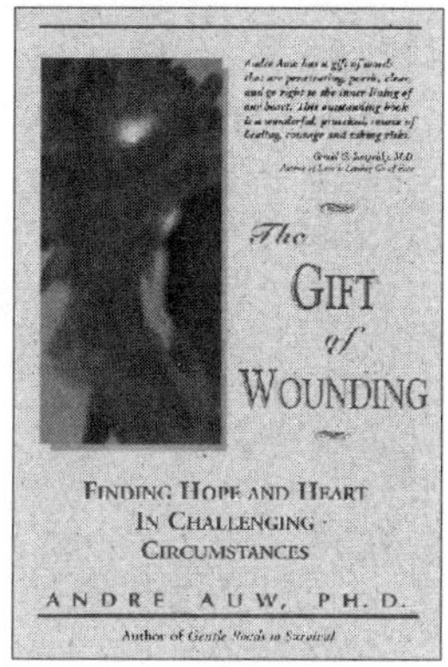

The Gift of Wounding: Finding Hope & Heart in Challenging Circumstances
by Andre Auw Ph.D.
$13.95
ISBN 0-944031-79-X

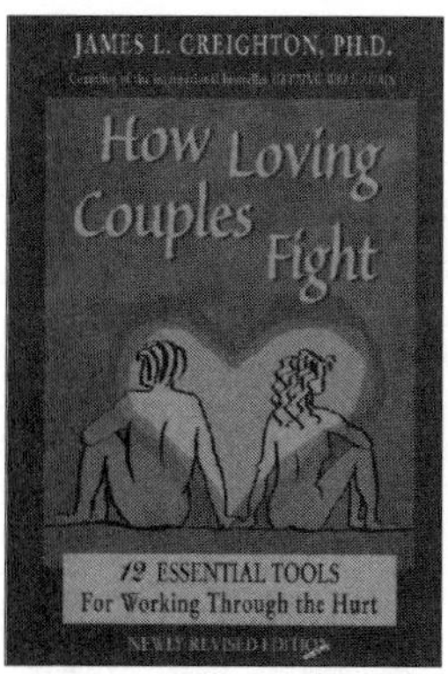

How Loving Couples Fight: 12 Essential Tools for Working Through the Hurt
by James L Creighton Ph.D.
$16.95
ISBN 0-944031-71-4

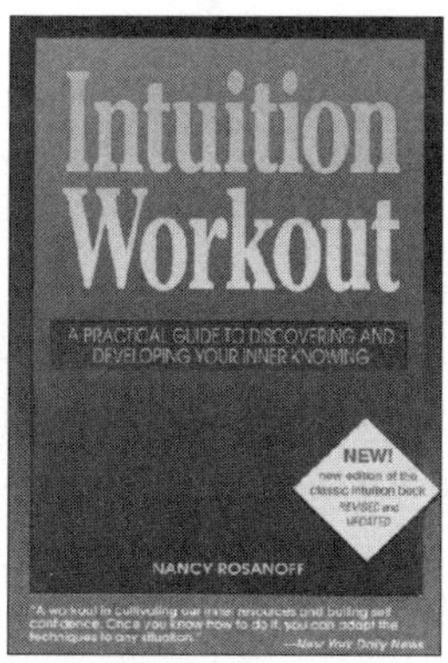

Intuition Workout: A Practical Guide To Discovering & Developing Your Inner Knowing
by Nancy Rosanoff
$12.95
ISBN 0-944031-14-5

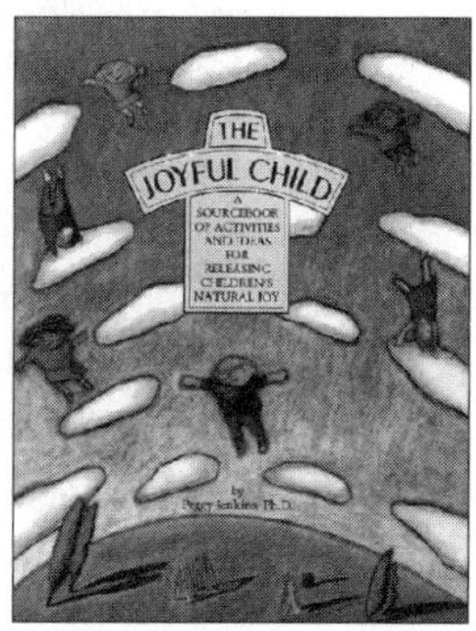

The Joyful Child: A Sourcebook of Activities and Ideas for Releasing Children's Natural Joy
by Peggy Jenkins Ph.D.
$16.95
ISBN 0-944031-66-8

Sing and Change the World
By David Edward Dayton, $16.95; ISBN 0-944031-92-7

The Sacred Weave
By Marianne Franzese Chasen, $13.95; ISBN 0-944031-91-9

To order any of Aslan's titles send a check or money order for the price of the book plus Shipping & Handling

Book Rate $3 for 1st book.; $1.00 for each additional book
First Class $4 for 1st book; $1.50 for each additional book

Send to: ***Aslan Publishing***
2490 Black Rock Turnpike # 342
Fairfield CT 06825

To receive a current catalog: please call (800) 786–5427 or (203) 372–0300
E-mail us at: **info@aslanpublishing.com**
Visit our website at **www.aslanpublishing.com**

Our authors are available for seminars, workshops, and lectures. For further information or to reach a specific author, please call or email Aslan Publishing.